ECGs by Example

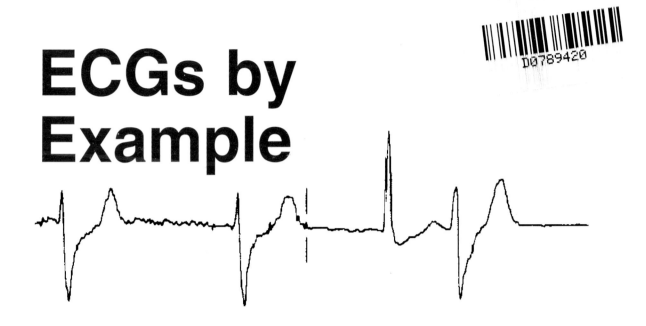

Richard Dean Jenkins

MB BCh MRCP

Medical Registrar
Royal Gwent and St Woolos Hospital
Newport
Wales

Stephen John Gerred

MB ChB

Medical Registrar
Waikato Hospital
Hamilton
New Zealand

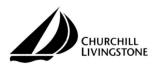

CHURCHILL
LIVINGSTONE

EDINBURGH LONDON NEW YORK OXFORD PHILADELPHIA ST LOUIS SYDNEY TORONTO 1997

CHURCHILL LIVINGSTONE
An imprint of Elsevier Science Limited

First published 1997
  Reprinted 1999
  Reprinted 2001
  Reprinted 2003

ISBN 0 443 056978

British Library Cataloguing in Publication Data
A catalogue record for this book is available from the British
Library

Library of Congress Cataloging in Publication Data
A catalog record for this book is available from the Library of
Congress

ELSEVIER SCIENCE   your source for books,
journals and multimedia
in the health sciences
www.elsevierhealth.com

Printed in China
C/04

The
publisher's
policy is to use
paper manufactured
from sustainable forests

'Real ECGs on the ward never look like the diagrams I've seen in textbooks.'

'I've read and understood the 'The ECG Made Easy' but I still get lost when confronted with the real thing.'

These are typical of the comments we have heard when trying to teach electro-cardiography to medical students, nurses and junior doctors. They are the reason why we have written this book. They are the reason why this book is different.

If you've read and understood an introductory ECG book, such as John Hampton's 'The ECG Made Easy', but still get phased by the real thing when it confronts you on the ward then this book is for you. All the examples are actual ECG recordings as they would appear in everyday practice. Each recording is at standard speed and size; 25 mm/sec, 1 cm/mV. We have endeavoured to include as many as possible of the commonly encountered abnormalities as well as some less common ECG findings which are of clinical importance. The content is based on a joint report by the American College of Physicians, American College of Cardiology and the American Heart Association (Fish C et al 1995 Clinical competence in electrocardiography. Journal of the American College of Cardiologists 25(6): 1465–1469). This report lists the electrocardiographic features that a competent physician should be able to recognise.

How to use this book
Each individual case consists of a full size ECG with a brief sentence summarising the patient's clinical presentation. Below each ECG there is a critique starting with a list of diagnostic features, then a full report of the ECG and any other clinical details that may be important. On most pages there is also a box of common causes or associations. You may wish to read the book as a text, use it to test yourself and others, or simply use it for reference purposes.

Becoming competent at interpreting real ECGs depends on seeing as many examples as possible and discussing them with a senior colleague. You may wish to use this book as a guide to building a comprehensive ECG collection of your own.

1997   RDJ
                                                    SJG

ACKNOWLEDGEMENTS

Our special thanks go to Dr Hugh McAlister, Cardiologist and electrophysiologist, and Dr Hamish Charleson, Cardiologist, both of Waikato Hospital, Hamilton, New Zealand. Without their help and guidance this book would not have been possible.

We would also like to thank all those who have helped us in the search of the more elusive recordings particularly: Dr Marjory Vanderpyl, Accident and Emergency Department, Waikato; Mrs Carol Rough, ECG technician, Waikato; Dr David Nicholls, Wellington, New Zealand; Dr Gowan Creamer; Dr Walter Flapper, Auckland; Dr Yadu Singh, Senior Cardiology Registrar, Waikato Hospital; Dr Michael Belz, assistant professor of internal medicine, Medical College of Virginia; Dr Peter Williams, Rheumatologist, Newport, Wales; and the staff of the Coronary Care Units at Waikato Hospital, New Zealand and the Royal Gwent Hospital, Wales. We would also like to thank Mr Andrew Gerred for his help with the software and hardware required to produce this book. We want to thank all the readers of the Internet newsgroups sci.med and sci.med.cardiology and the visitors to our 12-lead ECG website (http://homepages. enterprise.net/djenkins/ecghome.html) for their support.

Finally, we would like to dedicate the book to Clare and Susan for tolerating our 'hot air'.

CONTENTS

SUPRAVENTRICULAR RHYTHMS

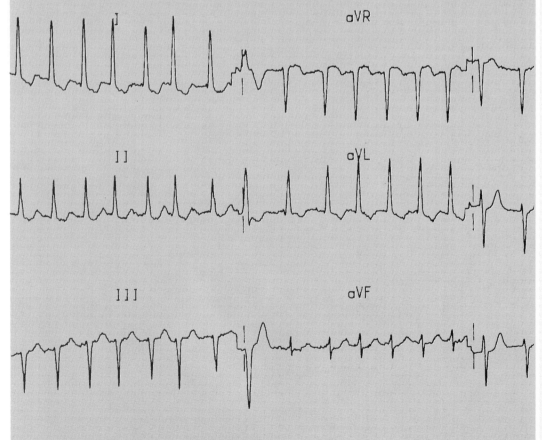

CASE 1

A 29-year-old healthy man

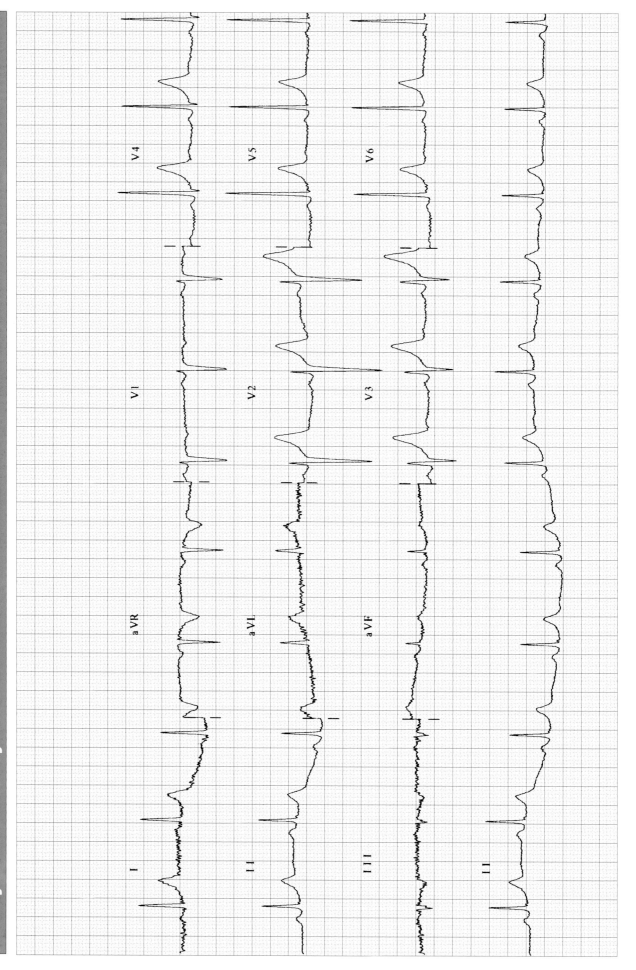

Normal sinus rhythm

- There are P waves.
- Each P wave is followed by a QRS complex.
- The rate is 60–100 b.p.m.

FEATURES OF THIS ECG

- Sinus rhythm, 66 b.p.m., normal QRS axis
- P waves followed by QRS complexes (Fig. 1.1)
- Baseline wander (Fig. 1.1)
  - the isoelectric line is not flat
- Skeletal muscle interference (Fig. 1.2)
  - high frequency irregular waves of muscular contractions

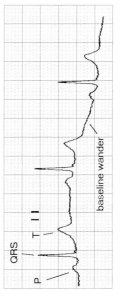

Fig. 1.1   Rhythm strip.

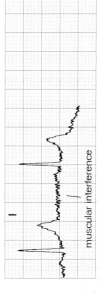

Fig. 1.2   Lead I.

Causes of poor ECG recordings

- ↑ Baseline wander
  - poor electrode contact, movement, twisted cables
- ↑ Skeletal muscle interference
  - anxious patient
- ↑ Electrical interference
  - poor insulation, poor filtering

CASE 2

A 25-year-old junior doctor

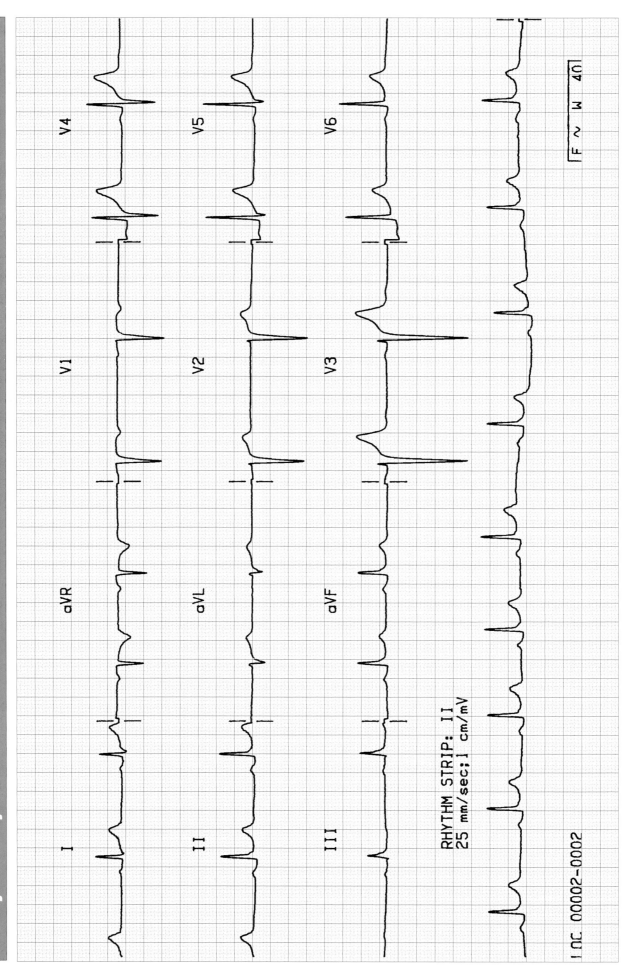

RHYTHM STRIP: II
25 mm/sec;1 cm/mV

Sinus arrhythmia (irregular sinus rhythm)

● A variation in the P–P interval of more than 10%.

Types of sinus arrhythmia.

1. respiratory – alternating periods of gradually lengthening and shortening P–P intervals (shown here)
2. non-respiratory
3. ventriculo-phasic – seen in association with complete heart block.

FEATURES OF THIS ECG

● Sinus arrhythmia, mean rate 54 b.p.m., normal QRS axis
● There are short P–P intervals at the beginning of the rhythm strip (Fig. 2.1.) and longer P–P intervals at the end of the rhythm strip (Fig. 2.2.)
● Early repolarisation in leads II, III, V5 and V6

CLINICAL NOTE

The cycle length is shorter (and the rate is faster) with inspiration.

Associations of sinus arrhythmia

↑ Seen in normal individuals
 – especially the young or athletic
↑ Accentuated by:
 – rest
 – digoxin
 – carotid sinus massage
↑ Abolished by:
 – exercise
 – atropine

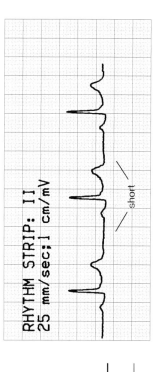

Fig. 2.1 Short cycles.

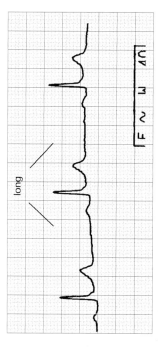

Fig. 2.2 Longer cycles.

CASE 3

A 60-year-old man with hypertension and angina

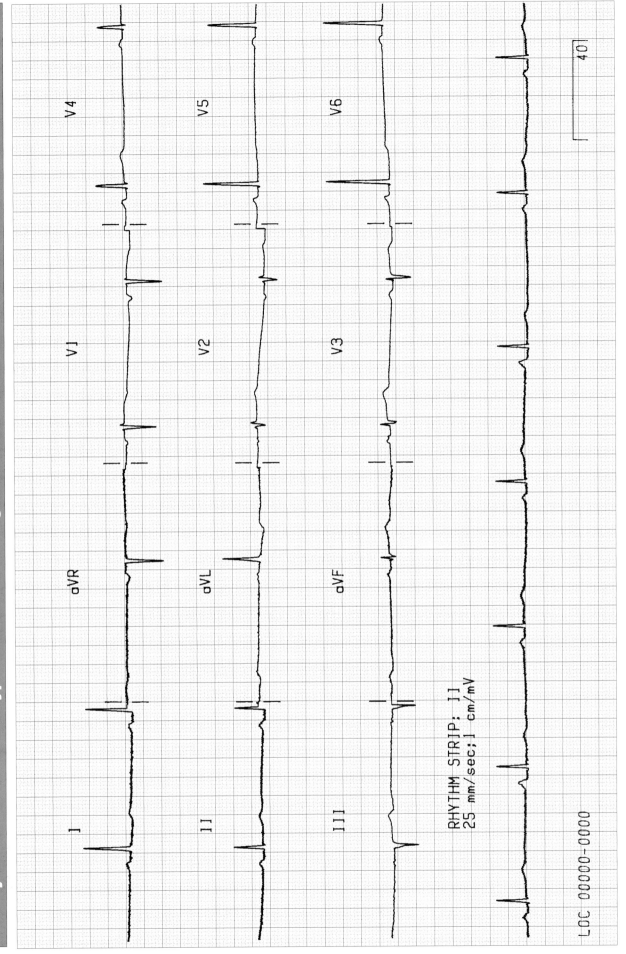

Sinus bradycardia

- Sinus rhythm with a rate less than 60 b.p.m.

- Beats 2 and 5 of the rhythm strip are atrial premature beats:
  - occur earlier than expected
  - preceded by an abnormal P wave

FEATURES OF THIS ECG

- Sinus bradycardia, 40 b.p.m., normal axis
- There is a slow P wave rate (Fig. 3.1)
- Incomplete right bundle branch block (Fig. 3.2)
  - an rSr′ pattern in V1
- Features suggesting left ventricular hypertrophy:
  - left atrial abnormality (Fig. 3.2)
  - non-specific lateral ST–T abnormalities
- A normal Q wave in lead III (Fig. 3.3)
  - although wide > 40 ms (1 small square), there is no q in aVF
    > 20 ms or q in lead II
  - normal Q waves in lead III disappear with deep inspiration

CLINICAL NOTE

This man was on a beta blocker.

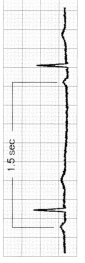

Fig. 3.1 Rhythm strip.

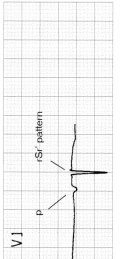

Fig. 3.2 Lead V1.

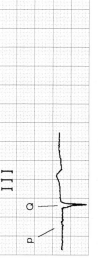

Fig. 3.3 Lead III.

Causes of sinus bradycardia

- ↑ Normal finding in athletes
- ↑ Sleep
- ↑ Drugs:
  - beta blockers, amiodarone
  - digoxin
  - calcium channel blockers
- ↑ Vasovagal syncope
- ↑ Sinus node dysfunction
- ↑ Hypothyroidism
- ↑ Obstructive jaundice
- ↑ Uraemia
- ↑ Increased intracranial pressure
- ↑ Glaucoma

CASE 4

A 73-year-old man with pneumonia

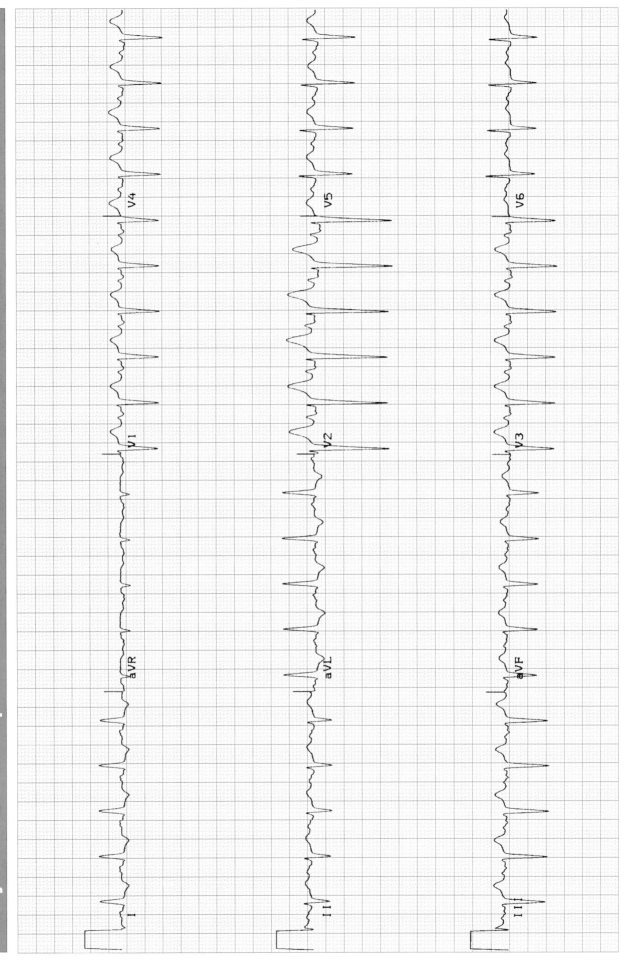

Sinus tachycardia

• Sinus rhythm with a rate greater than 100 b.p.m.

FEATURES OF THIS ECG

• Sinus tachycardia, 126 b.p.m., left axis deviation (−50°)
• There is a rapid P wave rate (Fig. 4.1)
• Left atrial hypertrophy (Fig. 4.1):
  – wide, notched P waves in lead II
• Left anterior hemiblock (Fig. 4.2):
  – left axis deviation
  – initial r waves in the inferior leads

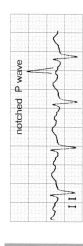

Fig. 4.1 P-mitrale.

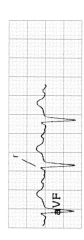

Fig. 4.2 Lead aVF.

Causes of sinus tachycardia

↑ Exercise
↑ Anxiety
↑ Fever
↑ Hypotension
↑ Cardiac failure
↑ Anaemia
↑ Pregnancy
↑ Thyrotoxicosis
↑ Pulmonary embolus
↑ Acute pericarditis
↑ Sinus node dysfunction

CASE 5

A 70-year-old lady with a stroke

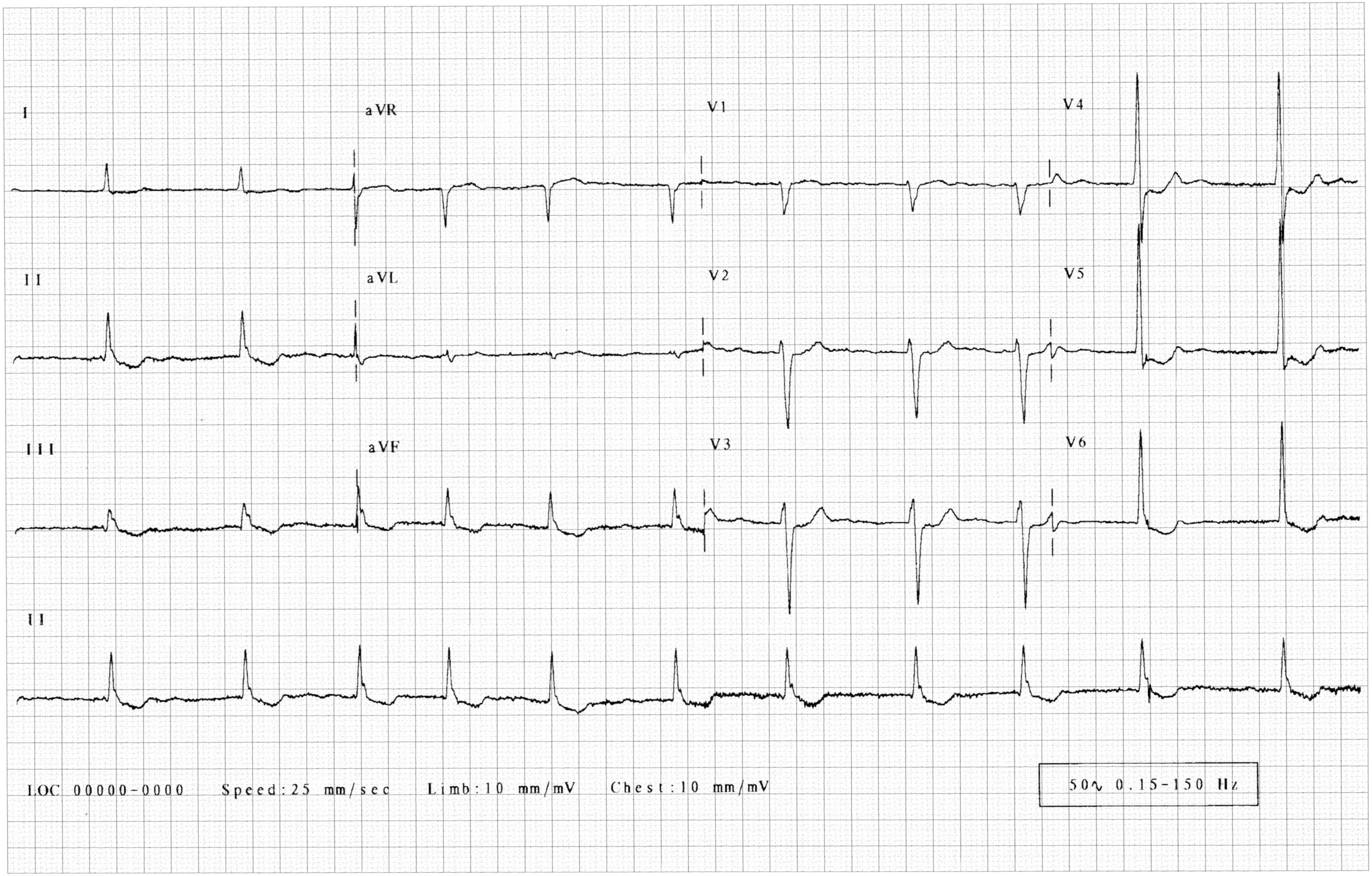

I

II

III

II

aVR

aVL

aVF

V1

V2

V3

V4

V5

V6

IOC 00000-0000   Speed:25 mm/sec   Limb:10 mm/mV   Chest:10 mm/mV

50~ 0.15-150 Hz

Atrial fibrillation

- There are no P waves.
- Fibrillary waves of irregular atrial activation may be seen.
- Ventricular response is irregularly irregular (random).

CLINICAL NOTE

This lady was taking digoxin, 125 μg daily.

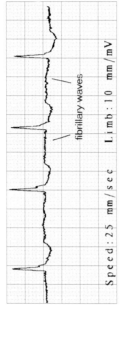

Speed: 25 mm/sec   Limb: 10 mm/mV

fibrillary waves

Fig. 5.1 Rhythm strip.

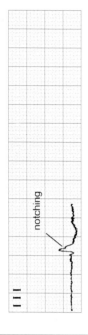

aVF

digoxin effect

reverse tick

Fig. 5.2 Lead aVF.

III

notching

Fig. 5.3 Intraventricular conduction delay.

FEATURES OF THIS ECG

- Mean ventricular rate 66 b.p.m., normal QRS axis
- Features of atrial fibrillation (Fig. 5.1):
  - no P waves
  - low amplitude, irregular fibrillary waves
  - random ventricular response
- ST segment changes consistent with digoxin effect (Fig. 5.2):
  - characteristic down-sloping ST depression (reverse tick morphology)
- Non-specific intraventricular conduction delay (Fig. 5.3)

Causes of atrial fibrillation

- ↑ Idiopathic
- ↑ Hypertension
- ↑ Mitral valve disease
- ↑ Cardiomyopathy
- ↑ Thyrotoxicosis
- ↑ Alcohol
- ↑ Sick sinus syndrome
- ↑ Cardiac surgery
- ↑ Autonomic
- ↑ Hypothyroidism
- ↑ Hyperkalaemia
- ↑ Sepsis

CASE 6

A 65-year-old lady with palpitations

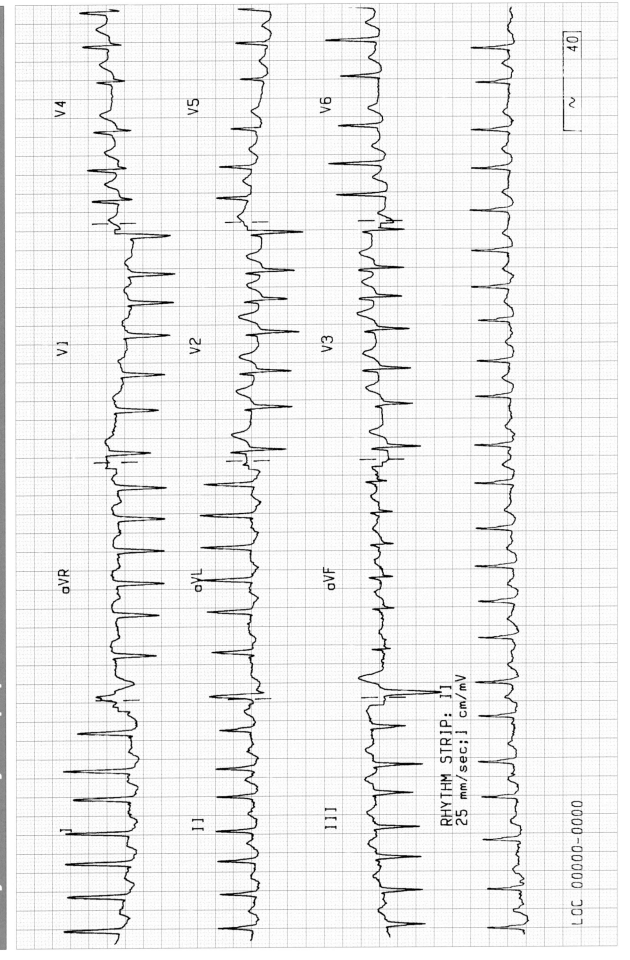

RHYTHM STRIP: II
25 mm/sec:1 cm/mV

LOC 00000-0000

Atrial fibrillation with rapid ventricular response

- There are no P waves.
- Ventricular response is irregularly irregular and fast.

FEATURES OF THIS ECG

- Mean ventricular rate 160 b.p.m., normal QRS axis
- Features of atrial fibrillation (Fig. 6.1):
  – no P waves
  – low amplitude fibrillary waves
  – random ventricular response – at first glance the rhythm looks regular but, on closer inspection, it is random
- Lateral ST–T changes (Fig. 6.2)
  – these often occur in tachycardia and are non-specific

CLINICAL NOTE

This lady had paroxysmal atrial fibrillation and was eventually controlled with oral flecainide.

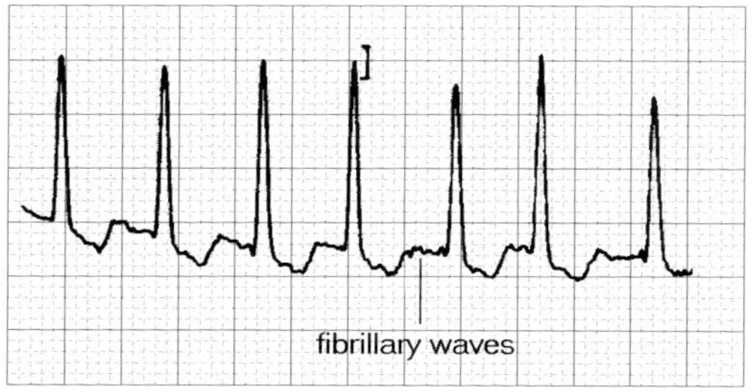

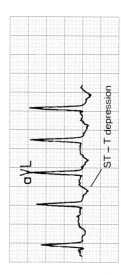

fibrillary waves

Fig. 6.1 Lead I.

aVL

ST – T depression

Fig. 6.2 Lead aVL.

CASE 7

A 55-year-old man with hypertension

I aVR V1 V4

II aVL V2 V5

III aVF V3 V6

II

Atrial flutter

- A characteristic sawtooth waveform seen in the inferior leads (flutter line) of a rapid atrial rate at 250–350 b.p.m.

Usually the atrial impulses are not all transmitted to the ventricles because of block in the AV node. Atrioventricular conduction often has a fixed ratio, e.g. 2:1, 3:1, 4:1 etc. (even commoner than odd), and sometimes a variable ratio producing an irregular rhythm.

Rarely 1:1 conduction can cause a very rapid tachycardia and may suggest an accessory pathway.

FEATURES OF THIS ECG

- Mean ventricular rate 72 b.p.m., normal QRS axis
- Atrial flutter with 4:1 AV block (Fig. 7.1):
  - the sawtooth wave is reproduced without the QRS complexes
  - the atrial rate is 288 b.p.m., exactly four times the ventricular rate
- Leads II and V1 are often good leads to see the rapid atrial rate (Fig. 7.2)

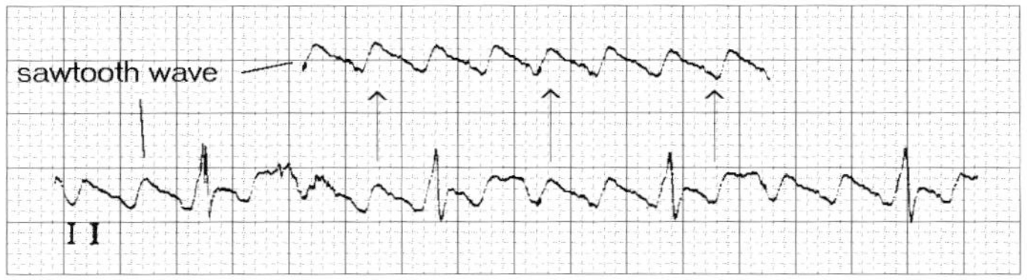

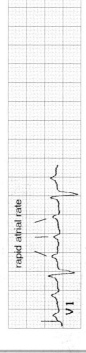

sawtooth wave

II

Fig. 7.1   Rhythm strip.

rapid atrial rate

V1

Fig. 7.2   Lead V1.

Causes of atrial flutter

→ Idiopathic
→ Ischaemic heart disease
→ Systemic hypertension
→ Valvular heart disease
→ Cor pulmonale
→ Cardiomyopathy
→ Thryotoxicosis
→ Congenital heart disease

CASE 8

A 79-year-old lady with dyspnoea and sweating

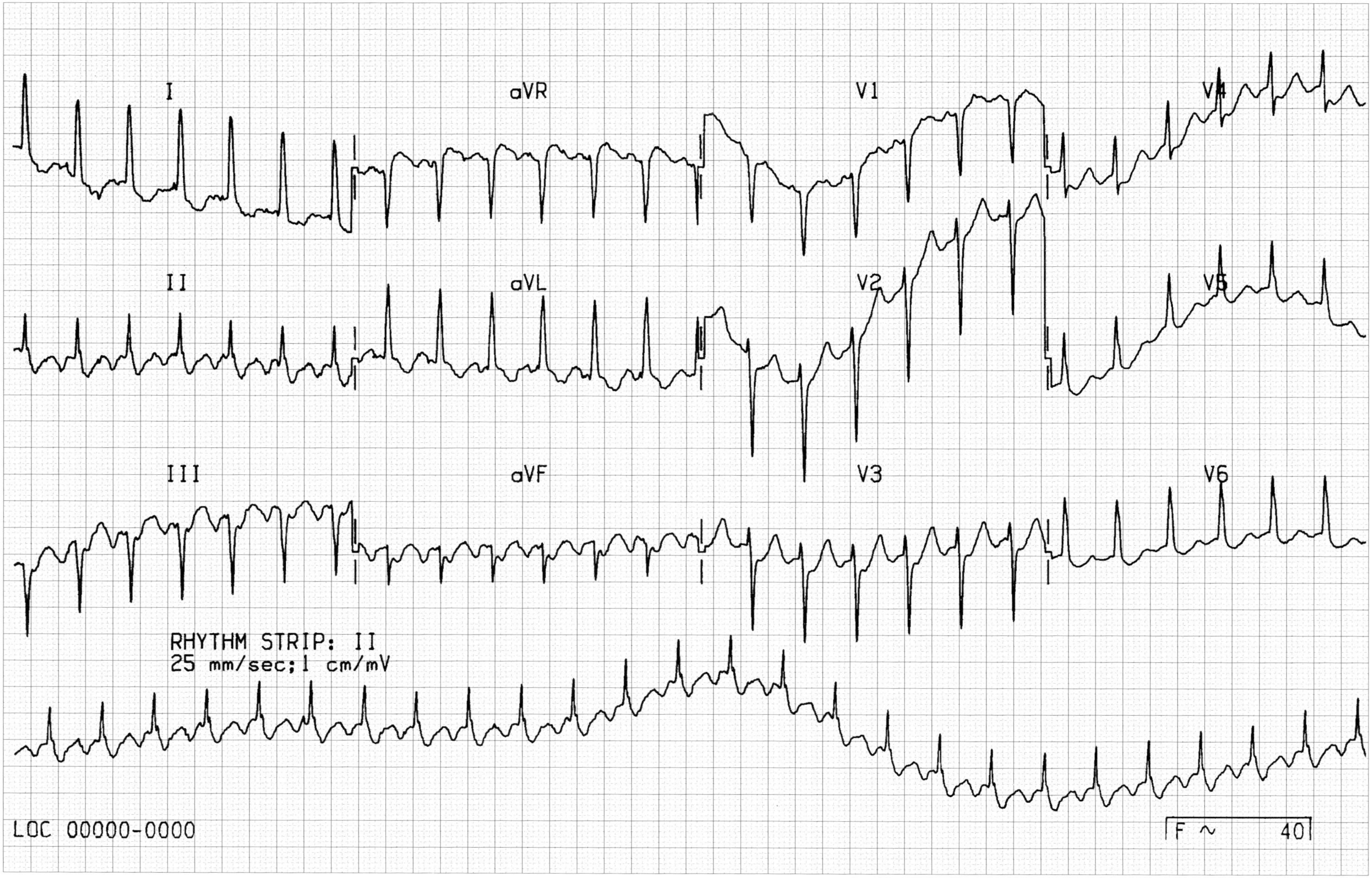

I

aVR

V1

V4

II

aVL

V2

V5

III

aVF

V3

V6

RHYTHM STRIP: II
25 mm/sec; 1 cm/mV

F ~   40

LOC 00000-0000

Atrial flutter with 2:1 AV block

Atrial flutter with 2:1 block is harder to see than higher grades of block.

● What gives it away is the rate of around 150 b.p.m. and a flutter line which can usually be found in one or more of the leads. Sometimes turning the whole ECG upside down will reveal the characteristic sawtooth wave.

FEATURES OF THIS ECG

● Mean ventricular rate 156 b.p.m., leftward QRS axis
● Atrial flutter with 2:1 AV block (Fig. 8.1):
  – distinct flutter line
  – the QRS rate is half the flutter rate
● There is a lot of baseline wander

CLINICAL NOTE

This lady had troublesome symptoms which were resistant to medical therapy. Attacks were prevented by disrupting the large intra-atrial re-entry circuit with radiofrequency ablation.

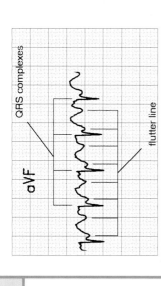

Fig. 8.1   Flutter line.

Clues to atrial flutter with 2:1 AV block

→ Obvious flutter line:
  – inferior leads and lead V1
  – ECG turned upside down
→ Episodes of higher grade AV block revealing flutter line:
  – spontaneous
  – carotid sinus massage
  – adenosine
→ Rate about 150 b.p.m.

CASE 9

A 50-year-old man with palpitations

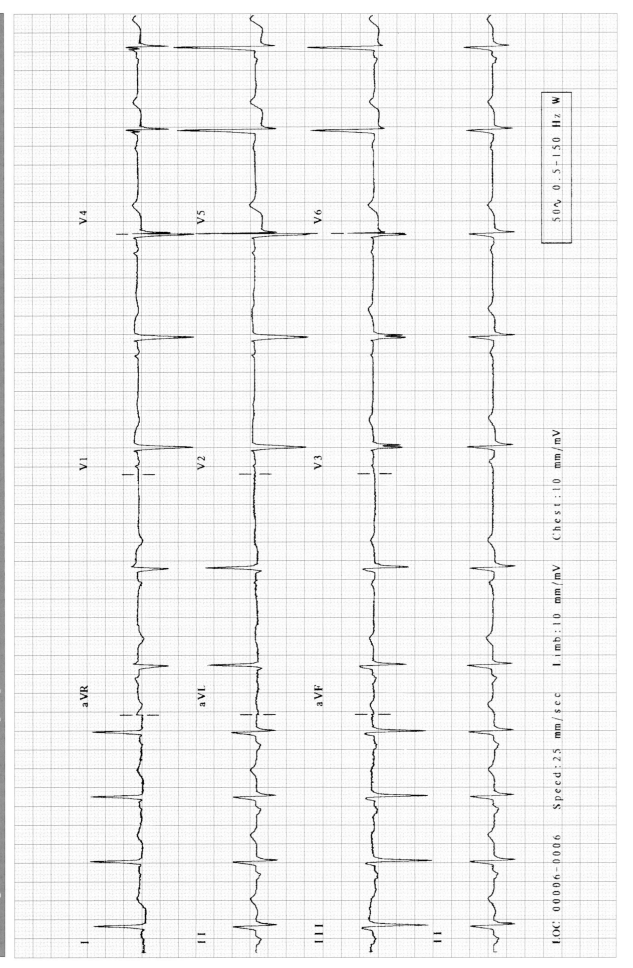

I

II

III

II

aVR

aVL

aVF

V1

V2

V3

V4

V5

V6

IOC: 00006-0006   Speed:25 mm/sec   Limb:10 mm/mV   Chest:10 mm/mV

50~ 0.5-150 Hz W

Ectopic atrial rhythm

An atrial pacemaker outside the sinoatrial node.

- A sequence of three or more atrial premature beats.
- Abnormal P waves.

FEATURES OF THIS ECG

- Two rhythms are present:
  - beats 1–5 and 11, ectopic atrial rhythm, 95 b.p.m.
  - beats 6–10, sinus bradycardia, 55 b.p.m.
- Leftward QRS axis
- Features of an ectopic atrial rhythm (Fig. 9.1):
  - abnormal P waves (p')
  - QRS morphology the same as in sinus rhythm
  - the pacemaker is probably low atrial
- Features suggesting systemic hypertension:
  - large voltage deflections (Fig. 9.2)
  - non-specific lateral ST changes (Fig. 9.2)

CLINICAL NOTE

This man had a long history of hypertension.

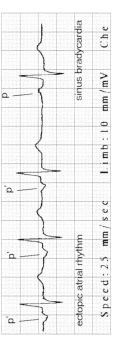

p' p' p' p p

ectopic atrial rhythm   sinus bradycardia

Speed: 25 mm/sec   Limb: 10 mm/mV   C:h:e

Fig. 9.1   Rhythm strip.

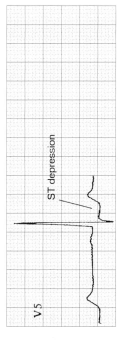

V5   ST depression

Fig. 9.2   Lead V5.

Common causes of atrial ectopic rhythm

↑ Sinus node dysfunction
↑ Any cause of structural atrial disease
↑ Ischaemic heart disease
↑ Electrolyte disturbance
↑ Drugs

CASE 10

A 65-year-old man with emphysema

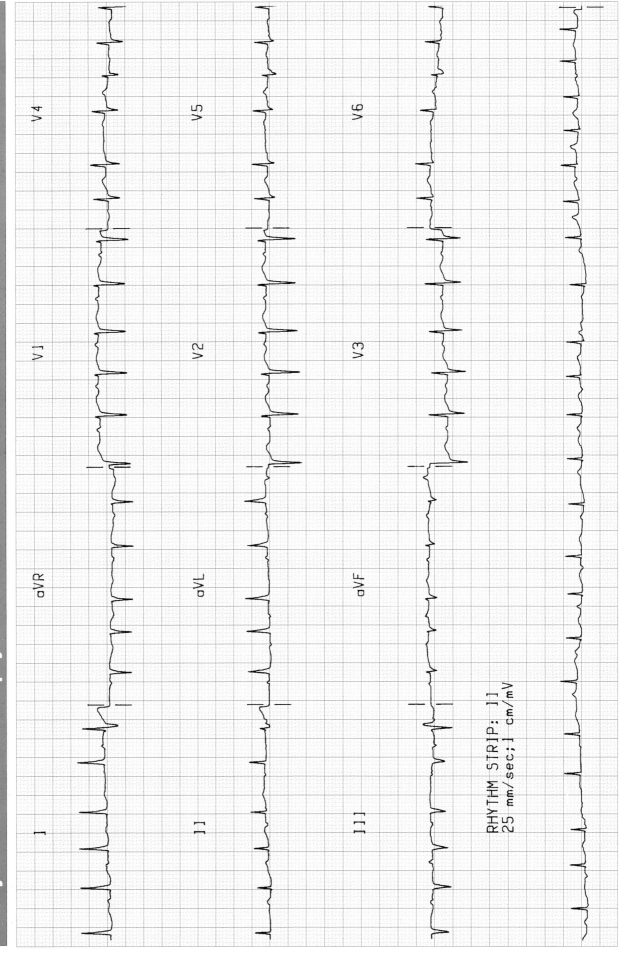

I

aVR

V1

V4

II

aVL

V2

V5

III

aVF

V3

V6

RHYTHM STRIP: II
25 mm/sec; 1 cm/mV

Multifocal atrial tachycardia

Multiple pacemakers outside the sinoatrial node.

- Irregular tachycardia, rate greater than 100 b.p.m.
- More than two P wave morphologies.

At rates below 100 b.p.m. this rhythm is often called 'wandering atrial pacemaker'.

FEATURES OF THIS ECG

- Mean ventricular rate 140 b.p.m., normal QRS axis
- Features of multifocal atrial tachycardia:
  - at least four different P wave morphologies (Fig. 10.1)
  - narrow complex, irregular tachycardia
- A normal Q wave in lead III
  - although wide > 40 ms (1 small square), there is no q in aVF > 20 ms or q in lead II
  - normal Q waves in lead III disappear with deep inspiration
- The voltages deflections are all small (a feature of emphysema)

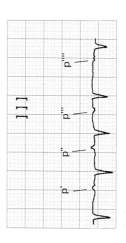

Fig. 10.1   Lead III.

Common causes of multifocal atrial tachycardia

↑ Chronic lung disease
↑ Ischaemic heart disease
↑ Alcohol

CASE 11

A 73-year-old lady 3 days after an episode of prolonged chest pain

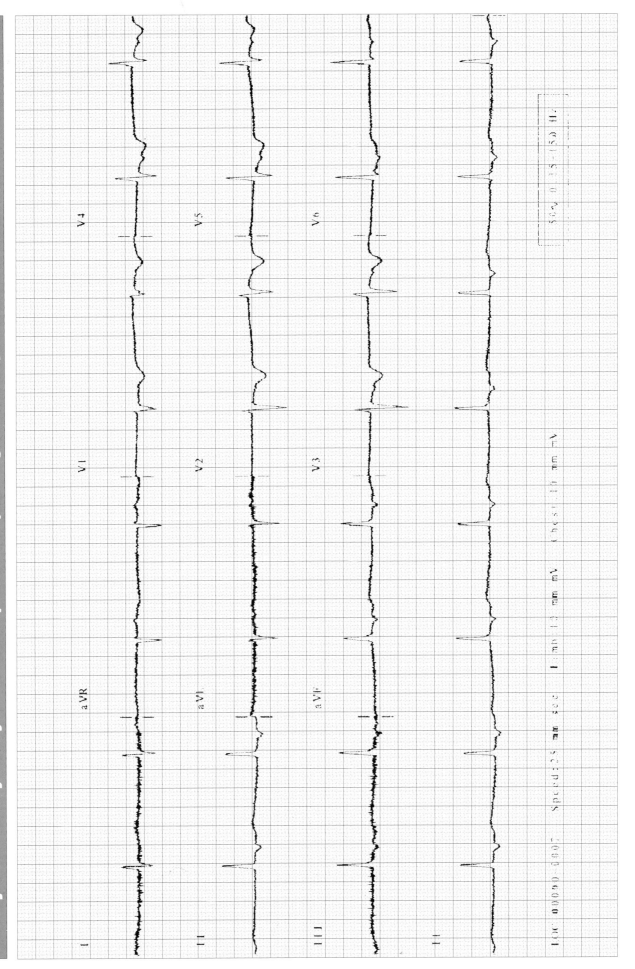

Junctional bradycardia

A sequence of three or more junctional escape beats at a rate less than 60 b.p.m.

- QRS complexes are the same as in sinus rhythm.
- P waves may be absent (sinus arrest), buried in the QRS, occur after the junctional escape, or occur as a result of retrograde conduction (inverted P wave).

FEATURES OF THIS ECG

- Junctional bradycardia, 48 b.p.m., normal QRS axis
- Junctional escape beats:
  - narrow QRS complexes with non-specific intraventricular conduction delay
  - inverted P waves seen following the QRS (Fig. 11.1) – shown to be distinct from T wave (Fig. 11.2)
- Changes suggesting ischaemia or subendocardial infarction:
  - abnormal ST depression and T wave inversion in the anterior leads V1–6
  - flattened T waves in other leads (Fig. 11.2)

CLINICAL NOTE

This lady had suffered a non-Q-wave myocardial infarction and was on a beta blocker.

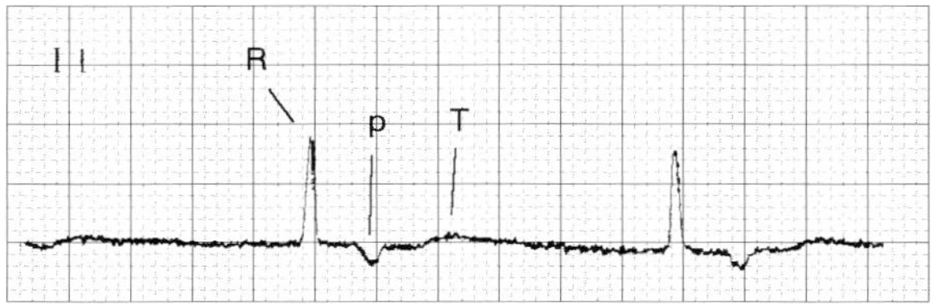

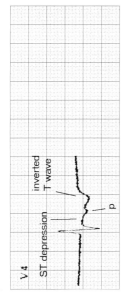

Fig. 11.1 Rhythm strip.

Fig. 11.2 Lead V4.

Causes of junctional bradycardia

↑ Normal finding in athletes
↑ Drugs:
  - beta blockers
  - amiodarone
  - digoxin
  - calcium channel blockers
↑ Sinus node dysfunction

CASE 12

A 26-year-old man with palpitations

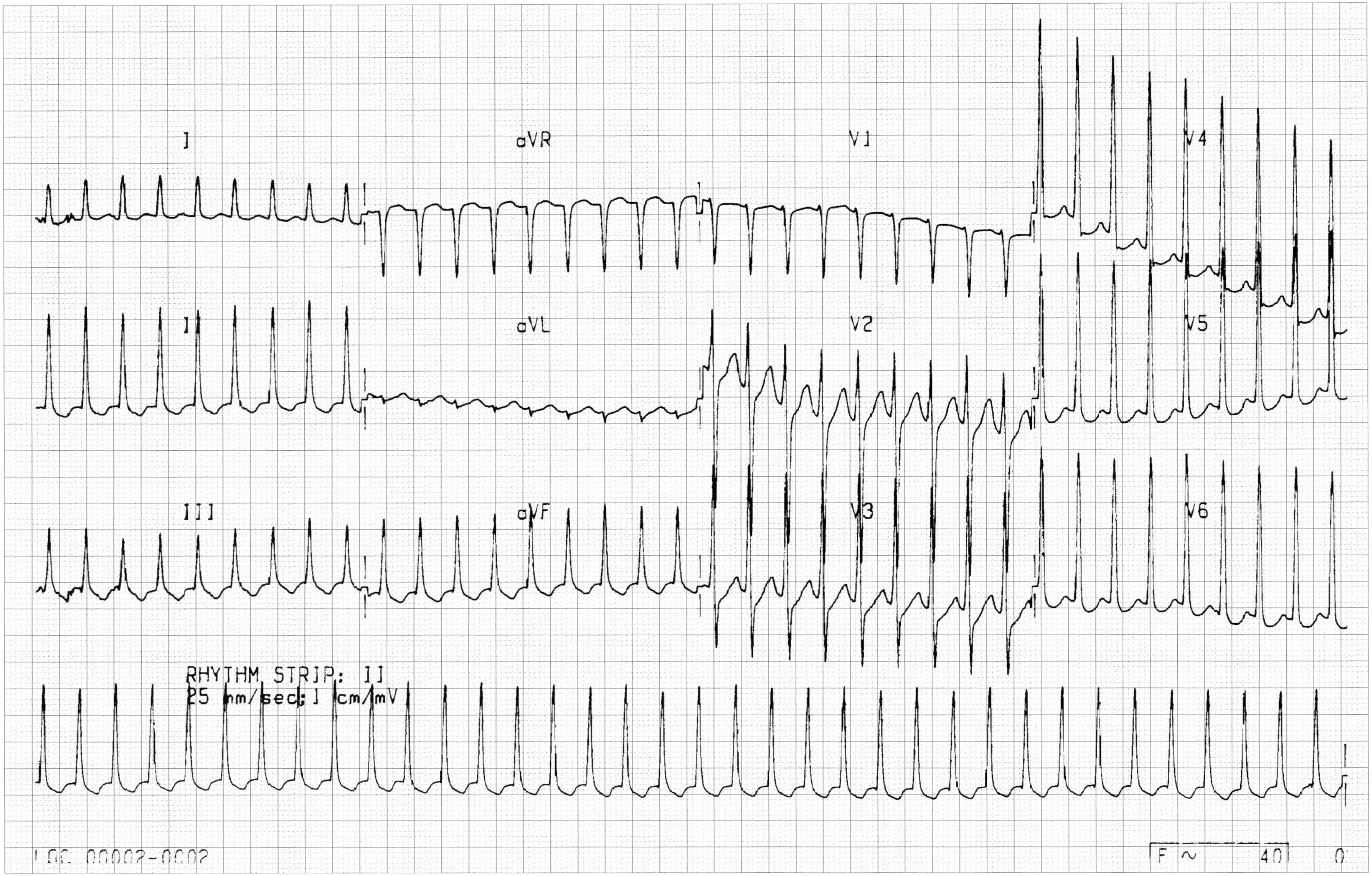
I
aVR
V1
V4
II
aVL
V2
V5
III
aVF
V3
V6
RHYTHM STRIP: II
25 mm/sec; 1 cm/mV
F ~ 40

Paroxysmal SVT – AV nodal re-entry tachycardia

A re-entry circuit within the AV node produces a tachycardia with the following features:

- narrow complex tachycardia
- usually 140–180 b.p.m. but can be as fast as 250 b.p.m.
- no visible P waves in the majority of patients as they are hidden by the QRS complexes
- if the P waves are visible then they are usually inverted and seen just after or (rarely) just before the QRS.

It is sometimes impossible to differentiate between AV nodal re-entry and AV reciprocating tachycardia.

CLINICAL NOTE

Electrophysiological testing confirmed the diagnosis of AV nodal re-entry tachycardia.

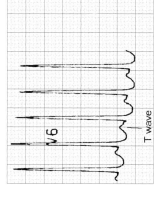

Fig. 12.2 Lead V6.

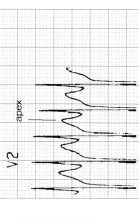

Fig. 12.1 Lead II.

Fig.12.3 Apex of T wave.

FEATURES OF THIS ECG

- Supraventricular tachycardia, 215 b.p.m., normal QRS axis
- Features of AV nodal re-entry tachycardia (Fig. 12.1):
  - regular narrow QRS complexes
  - no visible P waves
- T wave inversion and ST depression (Fig. 12.1)
  - this is often seen in tachycardia but is non-specific
- The apex of the T wave appears just prior to the QRS in the chest leads (Figs. 12.2 and 12.3)
  - do not mistake this for a P wave

Notes on AV nodal re-entry tachycardia

↑↑ Commoner in women than men
↑↑ Recurrent palpitations can be very distressing
↑↑ Fast and slow pathways within the AV node
↑↑ Radiofrequency ablation of the slow pathway is possible
  - greater than 95% success rate
  - risk of complete heart block less than 2%

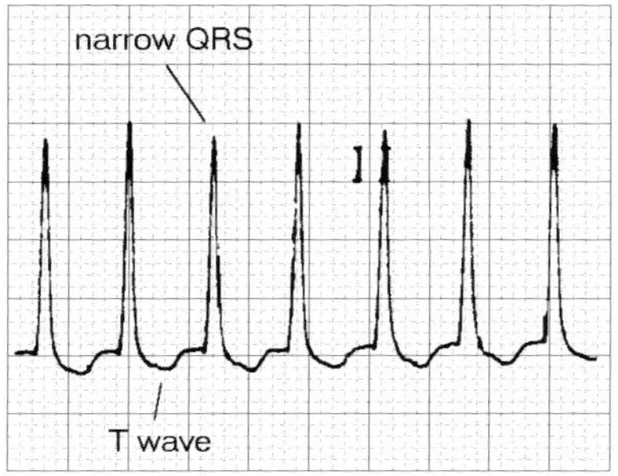

CASE 13

An 11-year-old boy with dizziness

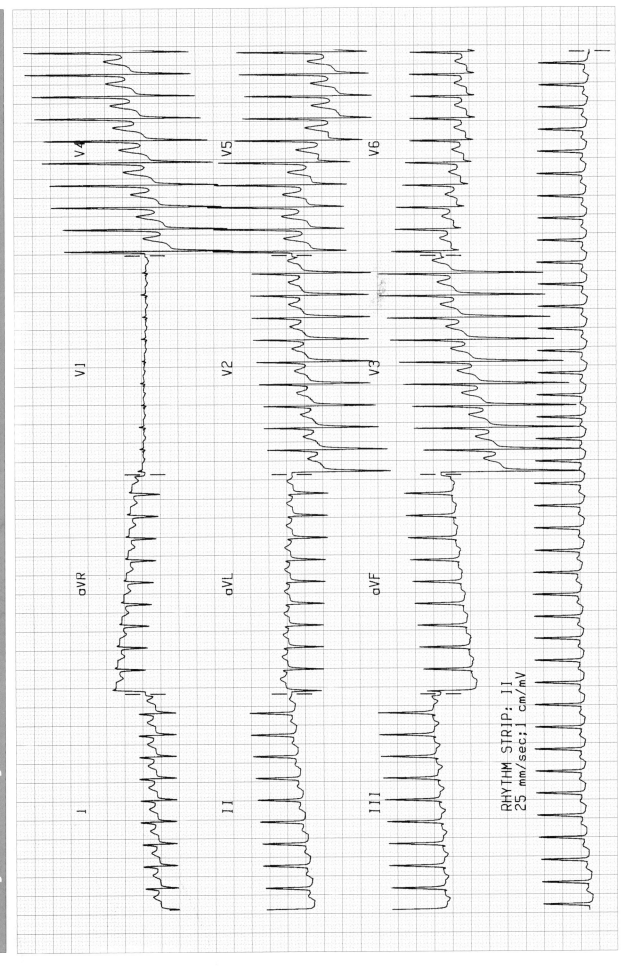

I

aVR

V1

V4

II

aVL

V2

V5

III

aVF

V3

V6

RHYTHM STRIP: II
25 mm/sec; 1 cm/mV

Paroxysmal SVT – AV reciprocating tachycardia (orthodromic)

A re-entry circuit from atria to ventricles via the AV node and returning to atria via an accessory pathway.

- Narrow complex tachycardia.
- Usually 160–250 b.p.m.
- The ECG in sinus rhythm may show a delta wave.
- P waves following the QRS seen more commonly than in AV nodal re-entry.
- Inverted P waves in the inferior leads and lead I are typical of a left-sided accessory pathway.

FEATURES OF THIS ECG

- Supraventricular tachycardia, 230 b.p.m., vertical QRS axis
- Features of paroxysmal SVT (Fig. 13.1):
  - regular narrow QRS complexes
- A possible P wave following the QRS complex (Fig. 13.2)
- ST depression (Fig. 13.3)
  - this is often seen in tachycardia but is non-specific

CLINICAL NOTE

The ECG after treatment with adenosine (p. 166) showed obvious delta waves supporting the diagnosis of AV reciprocating tachycardia due to Wolff–Parkinson–White syndrome.

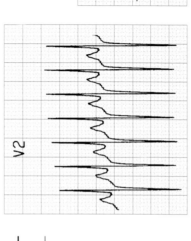

Fig. 13.1 Lead V2.

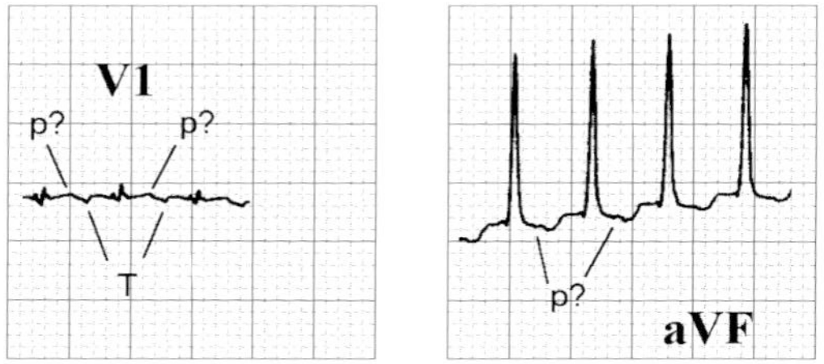

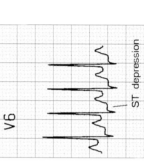

Fig. 13.2 P waves?

Fig. 13.3 Lead V6.

Notes on WPW-related tachycardias

↑ AV reciprocating tachycardias:
- orthodromic – commonest (shown here)
- orthodromic with aberrancy – wide complex
- antidromic – wide complex (pure delta waves), rare

↑ AF with rapid AV conduction

↑ VF

↑ Radiofrequency ablation is useful in symptomatic cases

CASE 14

A 13-year-old boy with recurrent bouts of tachycardia

AV reciprocating tachycardia (antidromic)

A re-entry circuit exists from the atria to the ventricles. There is antegrade conduction to the ventricles via an accessory pathway and retrograde conduction to the atria via the AV node.

- Regular, wide complex tachycardia.
- Usually 160–250 b.p.m.
- The ECG in sinus rhythm may show a delta wave with QRS morphology similar to the morphology during tachycardia.
- Typically, inverted P waves are seen between the QRS complexes.

FEATURES OF THIS ECG

- Wide complex tachycardia, 210 b.p.m., normal QRS axis
- Features of antidromic AV reciprocating tachycardia (Fig. 14.1):
  − regular, wide QRS complexes (pure delta waves)
  − inverted P waves between the QRS complexes

CLINICAL NOTE

After treatment the ECG in sinus rhythm (Fig. 14.2) showed a short PR interval, wide QRS complexes similar to those during tachycardia, a delta wave and secondary ST-T changes. This supports the diagnosis of antidromic AV reciprocating tachycardia due to Wolff–Parkinson–White syndrome.

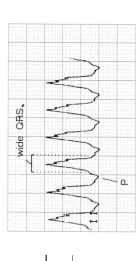

Fig. 14.1 Lead II in tachycardia.

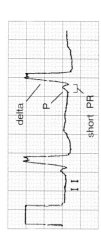

Fig. 14.2 Lead II in sinus rhythm.

CASE 15

A 16-year-old boy with recurrent faints

Wolff–Parkinson–White syndrome with atrial fibrillation

● Atrial fibrillation may be conducted rapidly to the ventricles when an accessory pathway is present. A wide complex, rapid tachycardia with an irregularly irregular rhythm occurs.

FEATURES OF THIS ECG

● Atrial fibrillation, 250–350 b.p.m., left axis deviation
● Typical features of WPW syndrome with AF (Fig. 15.1):
 – wide complex irregularly irregular rhythm
 – 'pure' delta waves
 – very short R–R intervals (shortest approximately 160 ms)
● There is a RBBB pattern (V1 positive)
 – this suggests a left-sided accessory pathway

CLINICAL NOTE

The resting ECG of this patient is shown on page 164.
The presence of pre-excited R–R intervals less than 260 ms (6.5 small squares), as shown here, increases the risk of ventricular fibrillation and sudden death.

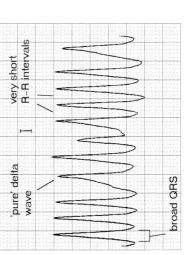

'pure' delta wave

very short R–R intervals

broad QRS

Fig. 15.1   Lead I.

Causes of wide complex, irregularly irregular rhythm

↑ AF with an accessory pathway
↑ AF with pre-existing bundle branch block
↑ AF with phasic aberrant ventricular conduction

CASE 16

A 48-year-old man with palpitations

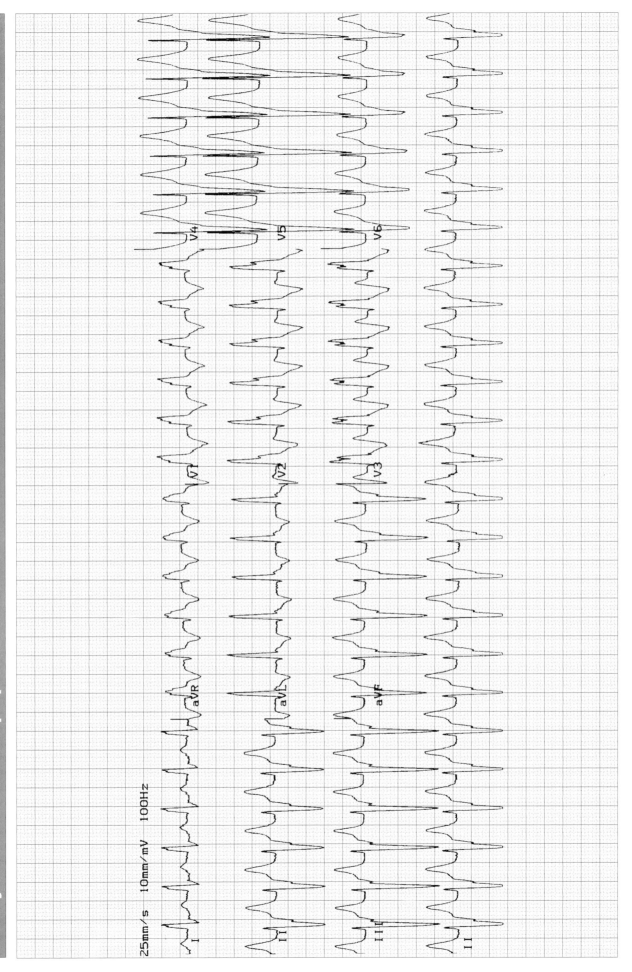

25mm/s   10mm/mV   100Hz

Supraventricular tachycardia with aberrant conduction

A wide complex tachycardia is VT until proven otherwise.[1]
No diagnostic criteria can differentiate all wide complex tachycardias.[2]

Factors favouring supraventricular tachycardia with aberrant conduction:

- the same morphology in tachycardia as in sinus rhythm
- irregularly irregular wide complex tachycardia
- R–S interval less than 70 ms (about 2 small squares)
- rSR′ pattern with R′ taller than r in lead V1
- converts with adenosine or carotid sinus massage.

- No fusion or capture beats
- A short R–S interval (Fig. 16.2)

CLINICAL NOTE

Adenosine was given and the rhythm converted to sinus rhythm with incomplete RBBB (Fig. 16.3). This suggests a diagnosis of paroxysmal SVT.

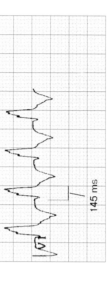

145 ms

Fig. 16.1   Wide QRS.

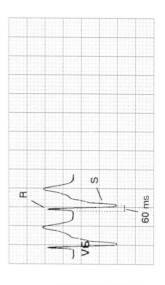

R

S

60 ms

V6

Fig. 16.2   R–S interval.

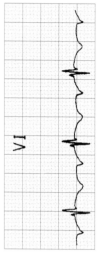

V1

Fig.16.3   After adenosine.

FEATURES OF THIS ECG

- Wide complex tachycardia, 144 b.p.m. (Fig. 16.1)
- Left axis deviation –60°
- RBBB with left anterior hemiblock pattern
- No AV dissociation is visible

Differential diagnosis of wide complex tachycardia

→ Ventricular tachycardia
→ Supraventricular tachycardia with phasic aberrant ventricular conduction
→ Supraventricular tachycardia with pre-existing bundle branch block
→ Wolff–Parkinson–White syndrome (antidromic tachycardia)

[1] Griffith M J, Garrat C J, Mounsey P, Camm A J 1994 Ventricular tachycardia as the default diagnosis in broad complex tachycardia. Lancet 343: 386
[2] Brugada P, Brugada J, Mont L et al 1991 A new approach to the differential diagnosis of a regular tachycardia with a wide QRS complex. Circulation 83: 1649–1659

CASE 17

A 48-year-old lady with blackouts

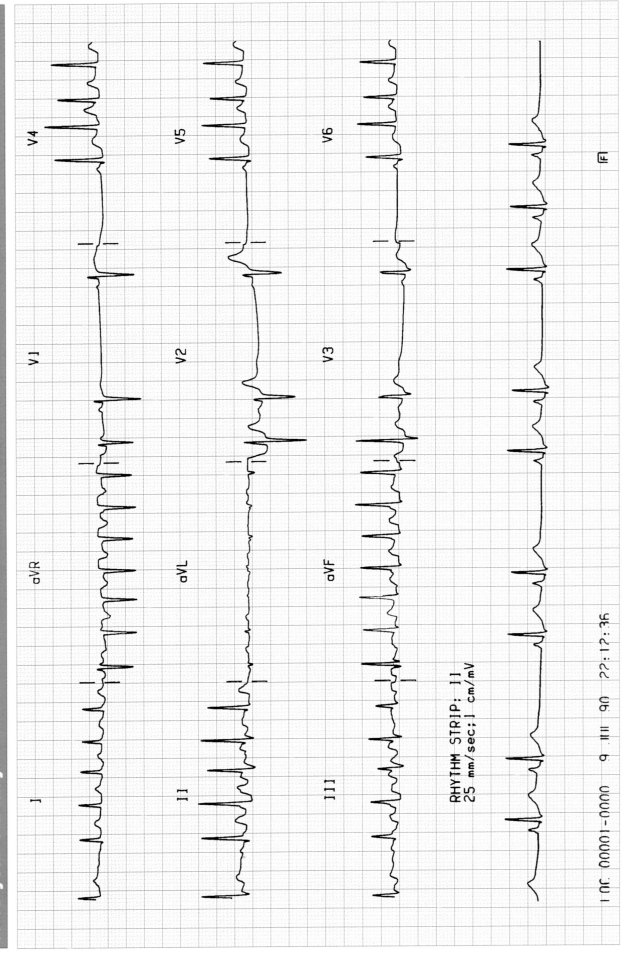

RHYTHM STRIP: II
25 mm/sec; 1 cm/mV

Sick sinus syndrome

Sick sinus syndrome is a term that covers a number of abnormalities including:

- spontaneous sinus bradycardia
- sinus arrest or sino-atrial exit block
- paroxysms of regular or irregular atrial tachyarrhythmias
- inadequate heart rate response to exercise.

FEATURES OF THIS ECG

It is very fortunate to have caught a number of the features of sick sinus syndrome on one 12-lead recording. Usually a 24-hour tape is required.

- Paroxysms of atrial fibrillation, rate 150 b.p.m. (Fig. 17.1)
  – with long secondary pauses on termination
- 3:2 sino-atrial exit block (Fig. 17.2)
- Normal QRS axis

CLINICAL NOTE

This lady had a florid form of sick sinus syndrome. On other occasions she had sinus pauses lasting 5–6 seconds with syncope, atrial flutter and multifocal atrial tachycardia.

Symptomatic sick sinus syndrome is the commonest indication for a permanent pacemaker.

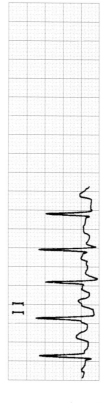

Fig. 17.1 Paroxysmal AF.

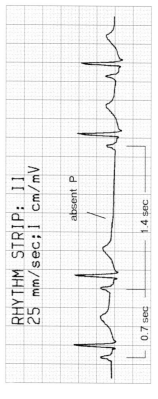

Fig. 17.2 Sino-atrial exit block.

VENTRICULAR RHYTHMS

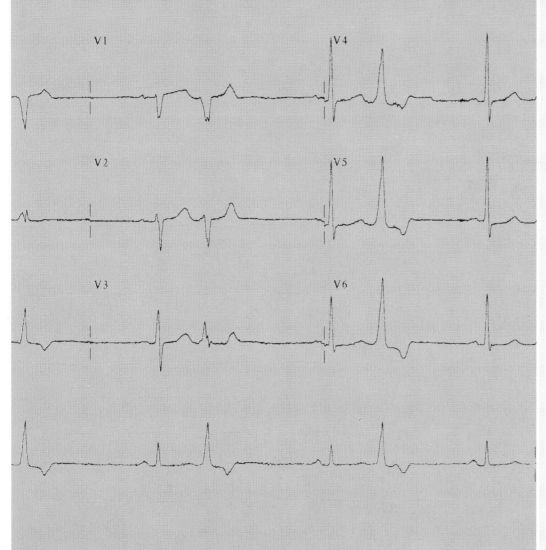

CASE 18

A 64-year-old man with irregular thumping sensations in the chest

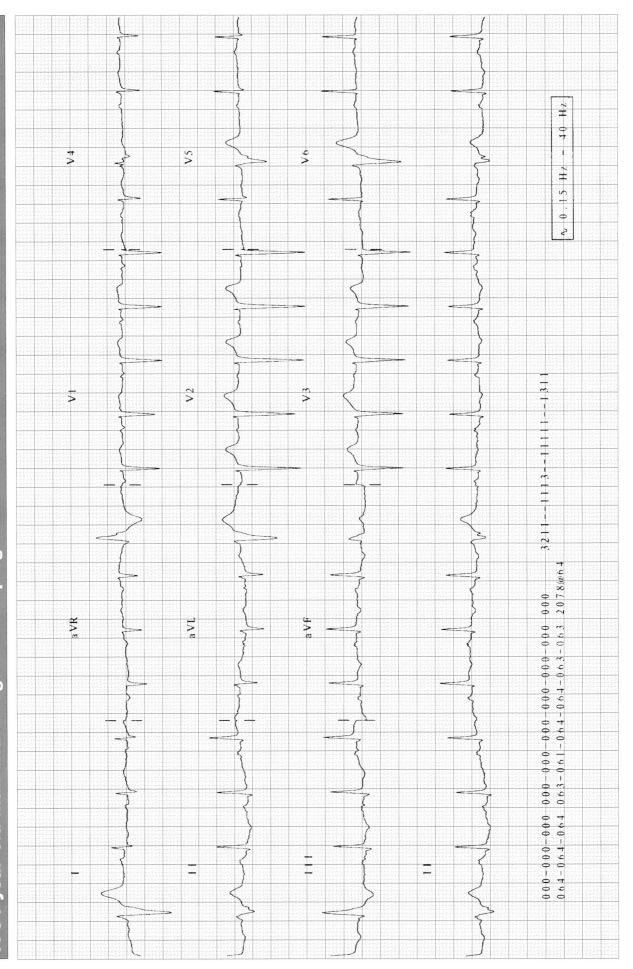

Ventricular premature beat (VPB)

- An abnormally wide beat occuring earlier than expected.
- There is no preceding P wave; AV dissociation is present.
- The premature beat is followed by a full compensatory pause, i.e. the R–R interval between the beats directly preceding and following the VPB is exactly twice that of the regular R–R interval.

P waves may often be identified in the T wave following a VPB, either as a result of retrograde conduction (P wave early and negative), or as dissociated sinus events (same P–P interval and morphology as the usual P wave).

When VPBs have different morphologies they are called multifocal.

FEATURES OF THIS ECG

- Sinus tachycardia, rate 105 b.p.m., normal QRS axis
- Ventricular premature beats (Fig. 18.1):
  – occur earlier than expected, no preceding P wave
  – abnormal shape, wider than sinus beats
  – followed by a full compensatory pause
- Abnormal Q waves in leads II, III, aVF suggesting an old inferior myocardial infarction
- Poor R wave progression in the anterior chest leads, consistent with an old anterior infarction

Common causes of ventricular premature beats

↑ Occur in normal individuals
↑ Ischaemic heart disease
↑ Digoxin toxicity
↑ Left ventricular dysfunction

CLINICAL NOTE

It is the normal beat following a VPB that is the more forceful and may cause a thumping sensation, not the VPB itself.

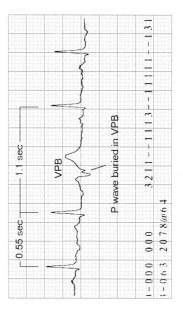

Fig. 18.1   Rhythm strip.

CASE 19

A 73-year-old lady with diabetes

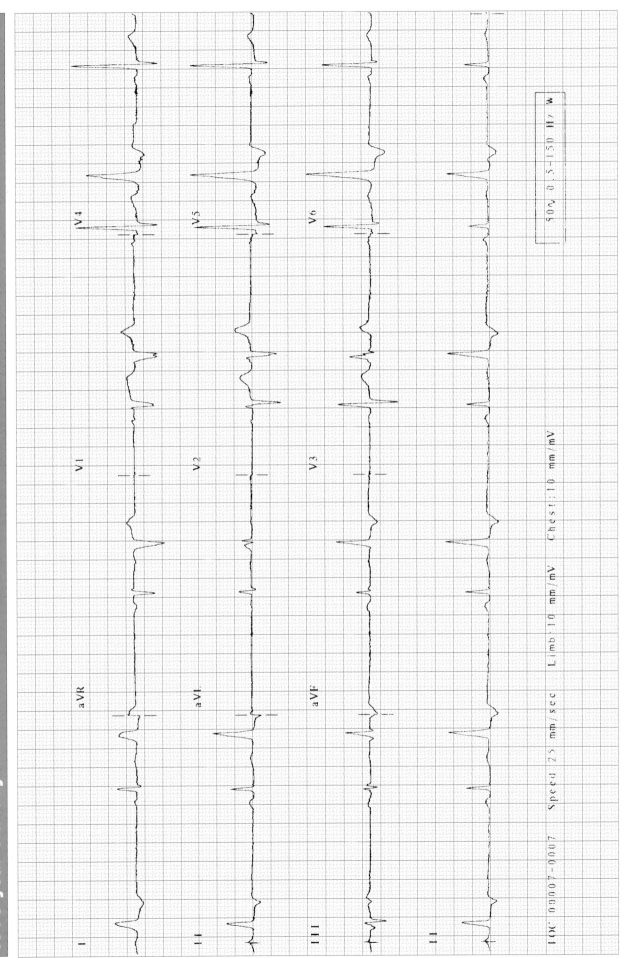

ICC 00007-0007   Speed 25 mm/sec   Limb 10 mm/mV   Chest 10 mm/mV

50∿ 0.5–150 Hz w

Ventricular bigeminy

- Each sinus beat is followed by a ventricular premature beat.
- The coupling interval is usually constant.

P waves may often be identified in the T wave of the ventricular ectopic beat, either as a result of retrograde conduction, or as dissociated sinus events.

FEATURES OF THIS ECG

- Sinus rhythm with ventricular bigeminy
- Atrial rate, 60 b.p.m. (every second P wave buried in the T wave of a VPB)
- Mean ventricular rate 60 b.p.m., normal QRS axis
- Ventricular bigeminy (Fig. 19.1)
  - Each sinus beat is followed by a ventricular premature beat (VPB)
- Non-specific intraventricular conduction delay
  - there is notching of the QRS complex in the sinus beats
- An artifact is present in leads II and III (Fig. 19.2)
  - such high frequency spikes should not be confused with pacing impulses

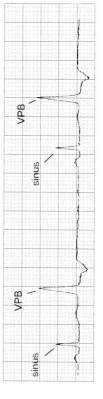

Fig. 19.1   Rhythm strip.

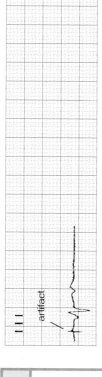

Fig. 19.2   Artifact.

Common causes of ventricular bigeminy

- ↑ May occur in normal individuals
- ↑ Ischaemic heart disease
- ↑ Digoxin toxicity
- ↑ Left ventricular dysfunction

CASE 20

A 78-year-old man 2 days following an episode of prolonged chest pain

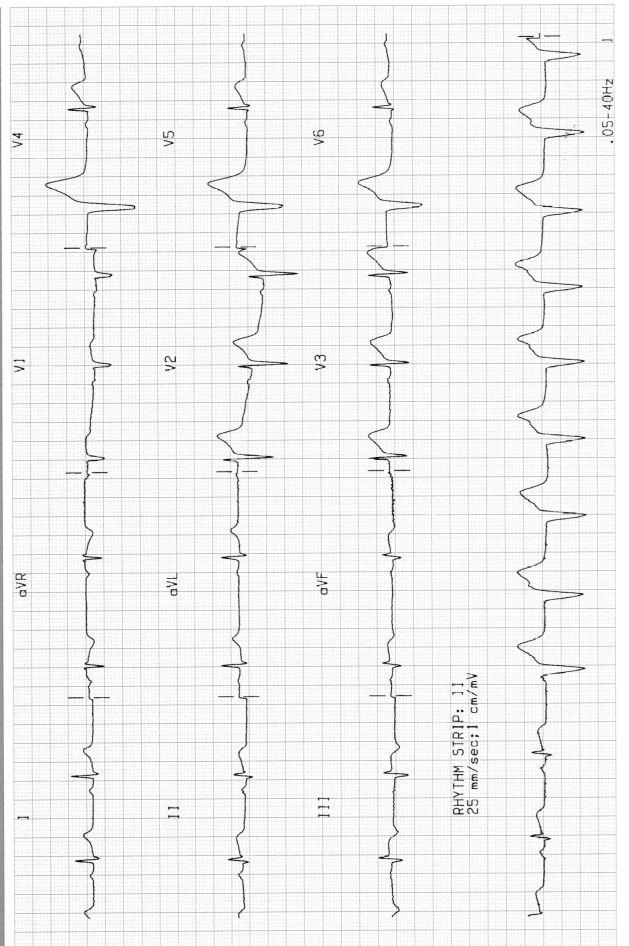

I

II

III

aVR

aVL

aVF

V1

V2

V3

V4

V5

V6

RHYTHM STRIP: II
25 mm/sec; 1 cm/mV

.05-40Hz

Accelerated idioventricular rhythm

- Wide complex regular rhythm, 60–100 b.p.m. (faster than sinus rate).
- Usually seen in association with an acute MI.
- It is thought to be a reperfusion arrhythmia.

P waves may often be identified in the T wave, either as a result of retrograde conduction, or as dissociated sinus events.

FEATURES OF THIS ECG

- Sinus rhythm, 60 b.p.m., normal QRS axis
- Accelerated idioventricular rhythm starts in the rhythm strip (Fig. 20.1):
  - wide complex, regular rhythm, 70 b.p.m.
  - P waves buried in the T wave (Fig. 20.1)
- Recent inferolateral myocardial infarction (Fig. 20.2):
  - abnormal q waves
  - ST elevation in leads II, III, aVF and V3–6
- A ventricular premature beat is recorded in leads V4–6

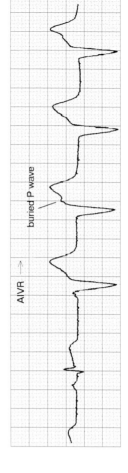

Fig. 20.1 Accelerated idioventricular rhythm.

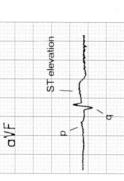

Fig. 20.2 Recent myocardial infarction.

Electrical origin of ventricular rhythms

→ Enhanced automaticity:
  - AIVR (shown here)
  - ventricular premature beats
→ Re-entry circuits:
  - ventricular tachycardia
  - ventricular flutter
  - ventricular fibrillation

CASE 21

A 55-year-old man, 2 weeks after a myocardial infarction, BP 130/80

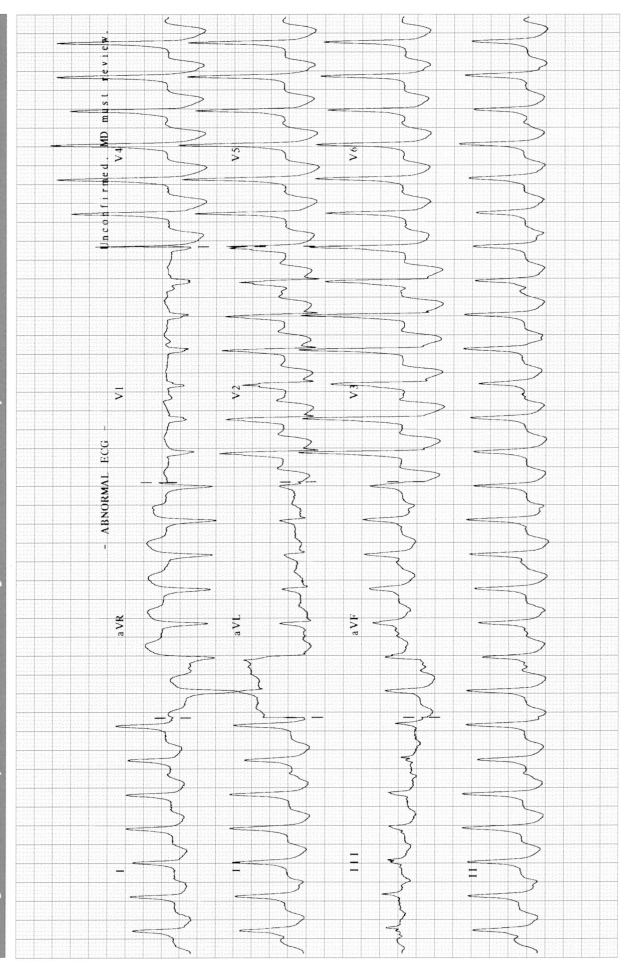

Ventricular tachycardia – atrioventricular dissociation

A wide complex tachycardia is VT until proven otherwise.[1]
No diagnostic criteria can differentiate all wide complex tachycardias.[2]

- Factors favouring ventricular tachycardia:
  – AV dissociation, fusion beats, capture beats
  – very wide complexes > 140 ms (3.5 small squares)
  – the same morphology in tachycardia as in ventricular premature beats
  – previous myocardial infarction
  – absence of any rS, RS or Rs complexes in the chest leads[2]
  – concordance – chest leads all positive or all negative.

FEATURES OF THIS ECG

- Ventricular tachycardia, 170 b.p.m., normal QRS axis
- Broad QRS complexes (Fig. 21.1)
- Obvious AV dissociation (Fig. 21.2)
  – AV dissociation is seen in less than 50% of cases of VT

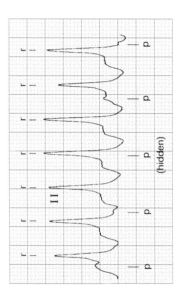

Fig. 21.1 Lead V2.

Fig. 21.2 Rhythm strip.

Causes of AV dissociation

→ Ventricular rate > atrial rate:
  – ventricular tachycardia
  – junctional tachycardia with retrograde block
→ Ventricular rate ≥ atrial rate:
  – sinus bradycardia with junctional escapes
  – accelerated idioventricular rhythm
→ Ventricular rate < atrial rate
  – second or third degree AV block

[1] Griffith M J, Garrat C J, Mounsey P, Camm A J 1994 Ventricular tachycardia as the default diagnosis in broad complex tachycardia. Lancet 343: 368
[2] Brugada P, Brugada J, Mont L et al 1991 A new approach to the differential diagnosis of a regular tachycardia with a wide QRS complex. Circulation 83: 1649–1659

CASE 22

A 24-year-old lady, previously well, with 6 hours of palpitations, BP 120/80

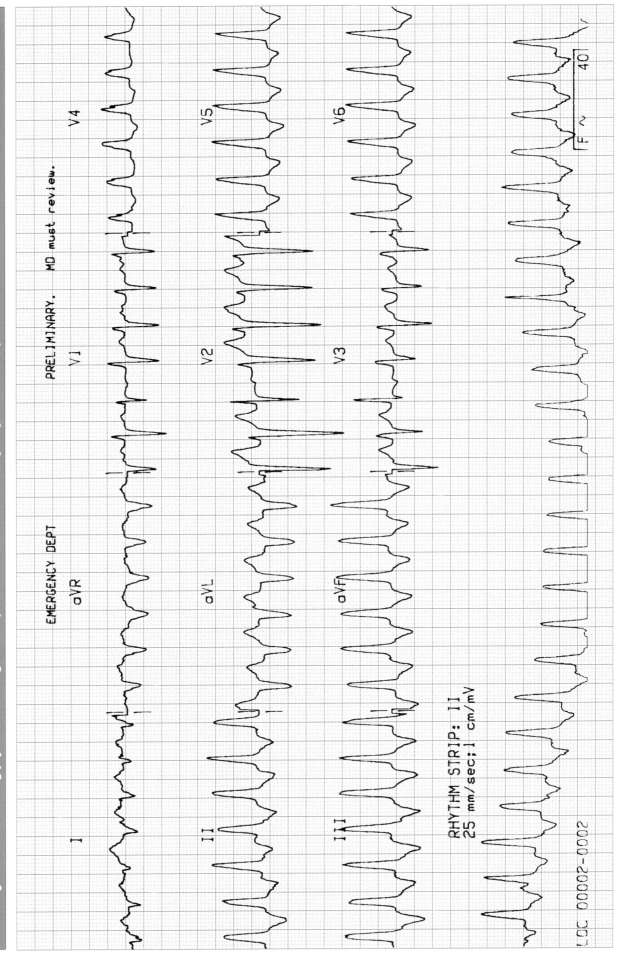

EMERGENCY DEPT   PRELIMINARY.   MD must review.

I   aVR   V1   V4

II   aVL   V2   V5

III   aVF   V3   V6

RHYTHM STRIP: II
25 mm/sec; 1 cm/mV

LOC 00002-0002

Ventricular tachycardia – capture and fusion beats

- A capture beat is a supraventricular impulse conducted to the ventricles in the middle of VT.
- A fusion beat is similarly conducted but coincides (and merges) with a ventricular impulse.

These are chance events and depend on critical timing. They are more commonly seen in VT with a slower rate and obviously in VT without retrograde conduction. Their presence strongly supports the diagnosis of VT.

FEATURES OF THIS ECG

- Ventricular tachycardia, 160 b.p.m., right axis deviation +100°
- Features favouring VT:
  - wide complexes and evidence of AV dissociation (Fig. 22.1)
  - a capture beat (Fig. 22.2) has the same morphology as in sinus rhythm (Fig. 22.3)
  - a fusion beat (Fig. 22.4) has a morphology in between sinus and ventricular
- Baseline wander of the rhythm strip

CLINICAL NOTE

This lady had catecholamine sensitive right ventricular outflow tract tachycardia and attacks have been prevented with a beta blocker.

Young age and no history of heart disease does not exclude a diagnosis of ventricular tachycardia.

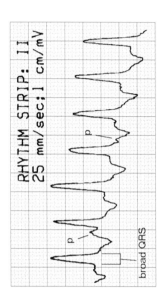

RHYTHM STRIP: II
25 mm/sec; 1 cm/mV

p
p
broad QRS

Fig. 22.1   Rhythm strip.

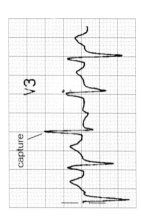

V3
capture

Fig. 22.2   Capture beat.

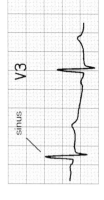

sinus
V3

Fig. 22.3   V3 in sinus rhythm.

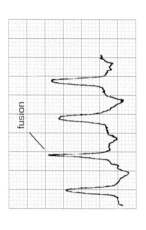

fusion

Fig. 22.4   Fusion beat.

CASE 23

An 80-year-old lady with ischaemic heart disease

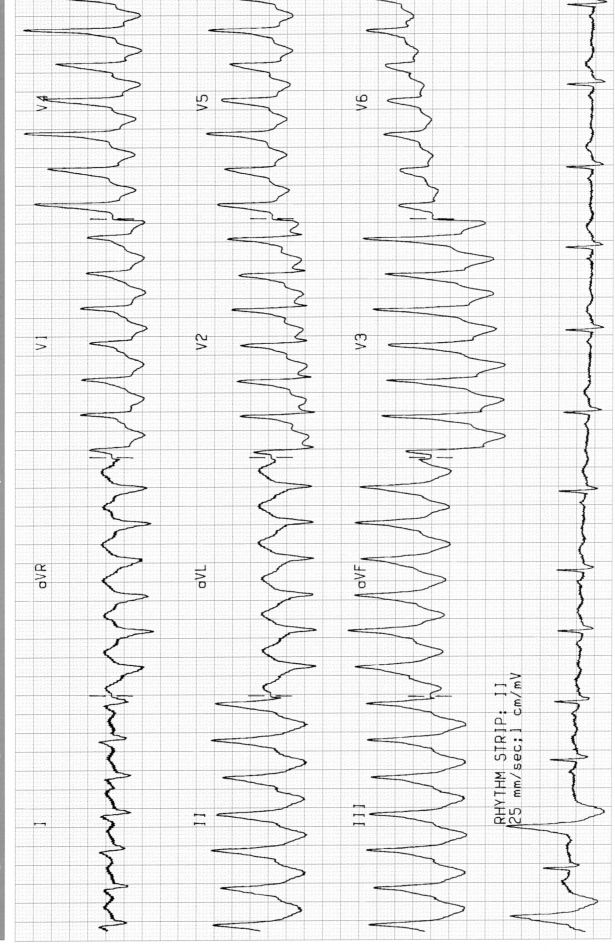

I   aVR   V1   V4

II   aVL   V2   V5

III   aVF   V3   V6

RHYTHM STRIP: II
25 mm/sec;1 cm/mV

Ventricular tachycardia – morphology of VPB

- When the morphology of a wide complex tachycardia is the same as that seen in ventricular premature beats (VPBs) then the diagnosis of VT is very likely.

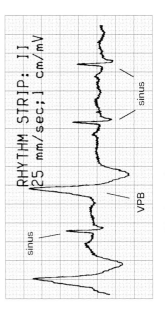

Fig. 23.1 Rhythm strip.

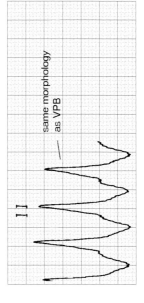

Fig. 23.2 Lead II.

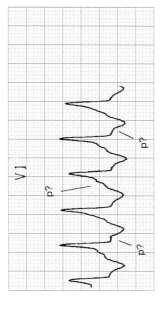

Fig. 23.3 Lead V1.

FEATURES OF THIS ECG

- Ventricular tachycardia, 160 b.p.m., axis +90°
- The rhythm has spontaneously reverted to sinus rhythm at the start or just before the rhythm strip
- A ventricular premature beat is seen in the rhythm strip (Fig. 23.1)
  - it has the same morphology as seen in the tachycardia (Fig. 23.2)
- There is a concordant pattern – all the chest leads are positive
- Atrioventricular dissociation is suspected (Fig. 23.3)
  - each complex has a slightly different morphology

CASE 24

A 66-year-old man with 'crushing' chest pain

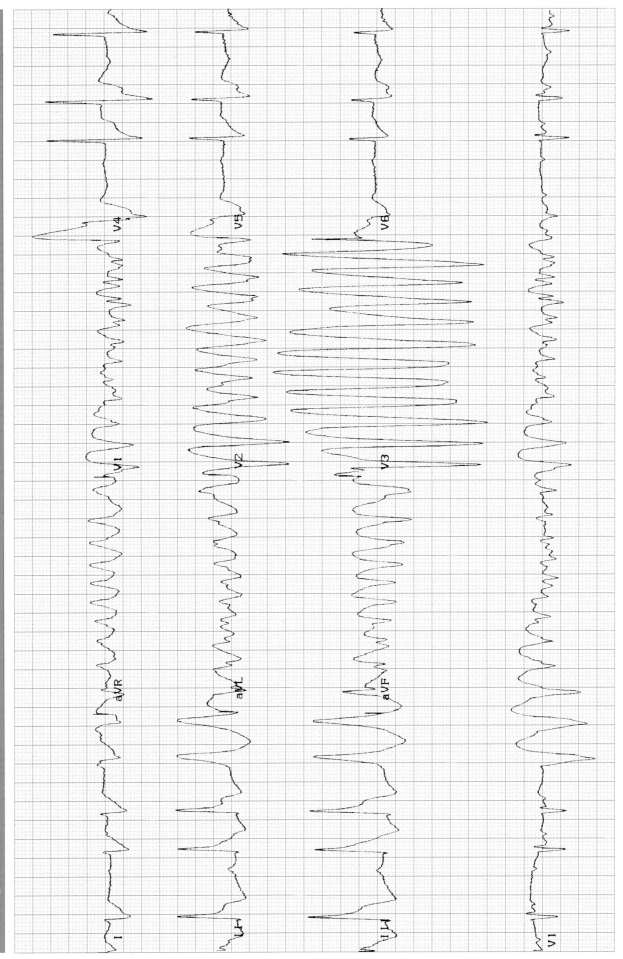

Polymorphic ventricular tachycardia

Polymorphic ventricular tachycardia is a form of VT in which there is usually no difficulty in recognising its ventricular origin.

- Multiple QRS morphologies, each beat usually differs from the previous one.
- Changing R–R intervals.
- Rate 150–300 b.p.m.

A particular type of polymorphic VT is 'torsade de pointes' and is shown on page 52.

- A burst, 6 seconds, of polymorphic VT (Fig. 24.3):
  – multiple morphologies
  – varying R–R intervals
  – mean rate 250 b.p.m.

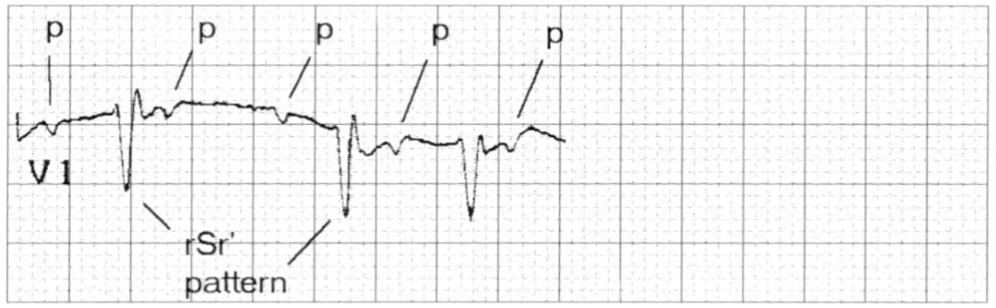

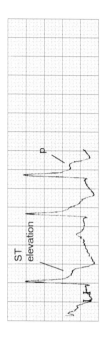

Fig. 24.1 Rhythm strip.

Fig. 24.2 Lead II.

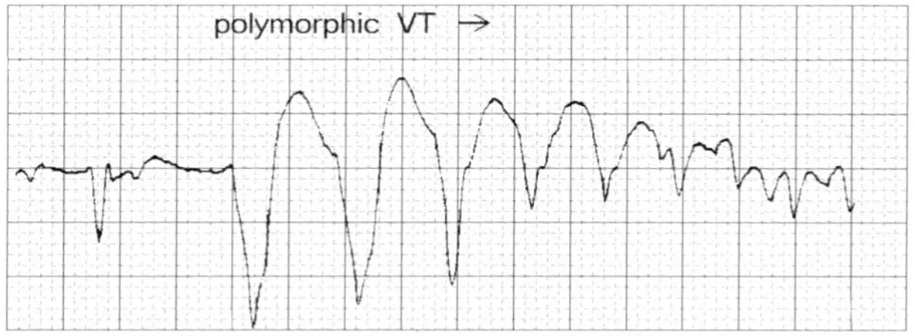

Fig. 24.3 Rhythm strip.

FEATURES OF THIS ECG

This ECG shows the advantage of a simultaneous rhythm strip recording
(note: in this ECG lead V1 has been used for the rhythm strip)

- Underlying rhythm (Fig. 24.1):
  – probably sinus rhythm with atrial ectopics
  – 80 b.p.m., right axis deviation, incomplete RBBB pattern
  – complete heart block
- Acute inferior myocardial infarction (Fig. 24.2):
  – ST elevation leads II and III
  – reciprocal changes (ST depression) in lead I, V4–6

Causes of polymorphic ventricular tachycardia

↑ Ischaemic heart disease, particularly acute infarction
↑ Impaired left ventricular function
↑ Long QT interval
↑ Electrolyte abnormalities
↑ Drugs
↑ Catecholamine sensitivity
↑ May occur in apparently normal hearts

CASE 25

A 35-year-old lady with blackouts

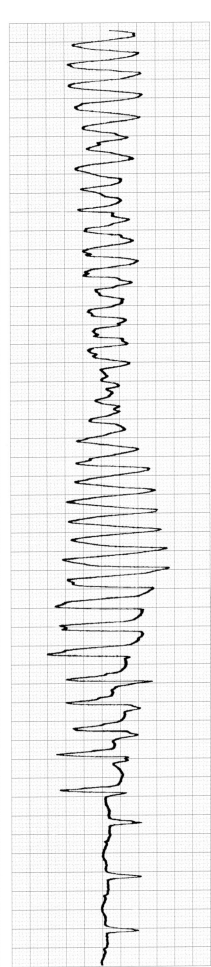

Polymorphic ventricular tachycardia – 'torsade de pointes'

A common form of polymorphic VT in which the axis seems to twist about the isoelectric line. (Torsade de pointes is a ballet term meaning 'to twist about a point'.)

The diagnosis of torsade de pointes is one of pattern recognition and is important as there are a number of reversible causes.

- The underlying sinus tachycardia has a prolonged corrected QT interval:
  - R–R interval = 560 ms
  - QT interval = 350 ms
  - corrected QT = 470 ms (normal less than 440 ms)

CLINICAL NOTE

This young woman was prescribed ketoconazole for a nail infection. During treatment she developed hayfever and purchased terfenadine from her local pharmacy.

FEATURES OF THIS ECG

- Torsade de pointes VT starts with an R on T phenomenon (Fig. 25.1)
  - a ventricular premature beat coincides with the T wave
- The morphology varies from beat to beat but in a characteristic repetitive manner

Fig. 25.1   Start of VT.

Causes of torsade de pointes tachycardia

- ↑ AV block
- ↑↑ Hypokalaemia
- ↑↑ Hypomagnesaemia
- ↑↑ Drug-induced long QT interval:
  - amiodarone, sotalol
  - class 1A antiarrhythmic drugs
  - tricyclic antidepressants
  - terfenadine in combination with ketoconazole/itraconazole
- ↑↑ Congenital long QT syndromes
- ↑↑ Other causes of a long QT interval:
  - IHD
  - subarachnoid haemorrhage
  - myxoedema

CASE 26

A 65-year-old man during an electrophysiology study (labels added)

Ventricular flutter

This is another form of VT which is characteristic for its rate and appearance.

- Very rapid, regular, wide complex tachycardia.
- Rate 300 b.p.m. or more.
- Sine wave morphology
- no distinction between QRS and T wave.

FEATURES OF THIS ECG

- Ventricular flutter, rate 300–340 b.p.m., left axis deviation
- Characteristic morphology (Fig. 26.1):
  - sine wave
  - no distinction between QRS and T wave
  - it is unclear where one complex finishes and the other starts
  - it looks the same if viewed upside down

CLINICAL NOTE

Ventricular flutter is usually short lived, associated with a marked fall in blood pressure and progresses to ventricular fibrillation.

This man was started on amiodarone and on retesting it was not possible to induce a sustained ventricular tachycardia.

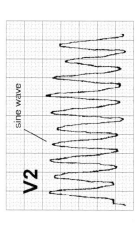

Fig. 26.1 Lead V2.

CASE 27

A 60-year-old man with chest pain and loss of consciousness

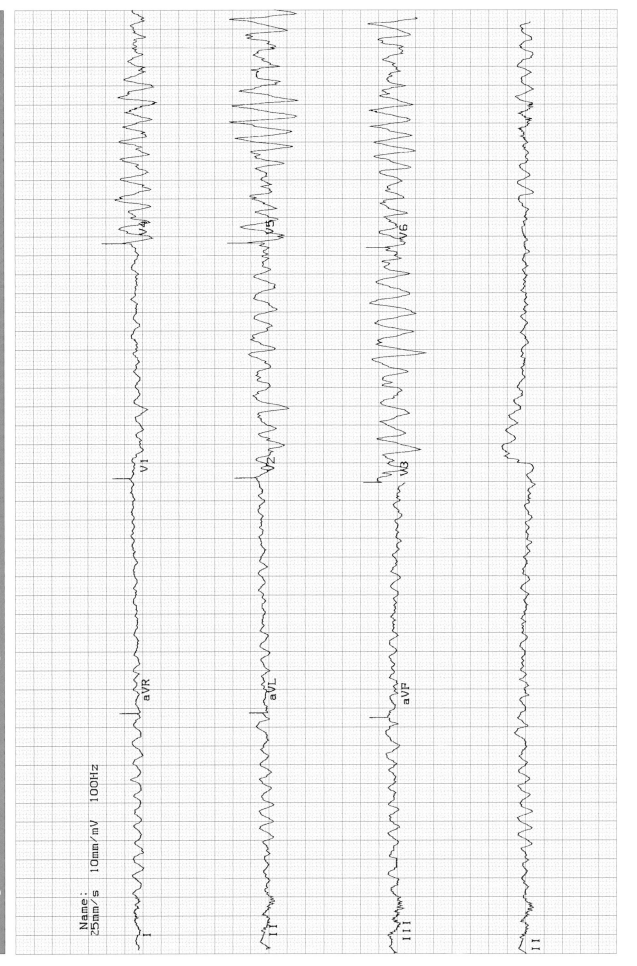

Name:
25mm/s   10mm/mV   100Hz

Ventricular fibrillation (VF)

- Totally disorganised and bizarre electrical activity.
- Undulating and unpredictable baseline.

FEATURES OF THIS ECG

- Ventricular fibrillation (Fig. 27.1)
- There is a pattern similar to torsade de pointes VT (Fig. 27.2)
  – VF consists of many foci of re-entry circuits; sometimes a pattern may form when one of these circuits becomes large but this is always short lived and localised

CLINICAL NOTE

This man collapsed during the recording! He was defibrillated, treated for a myocardial infarction and survived.

12-lead recordings of VF should never be taken, for obvious reasons!

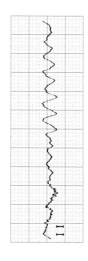

Fig. 27.1   Lead II.

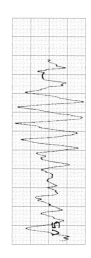

Fig. 27.2   Lead V5.

BUNDLE BRANCH BLOCK

Right bundle branch block (RBBB)

Incomplete right bundle branch block

Left bundle branch block (LBBB)

Incomplete left bundle branch block

Left anterior hemiblock

Left posterior hemiblock

Right bundle branch block with left anterior hemiblock (bifascicular block)

Phasic aberrant ventricular conduction

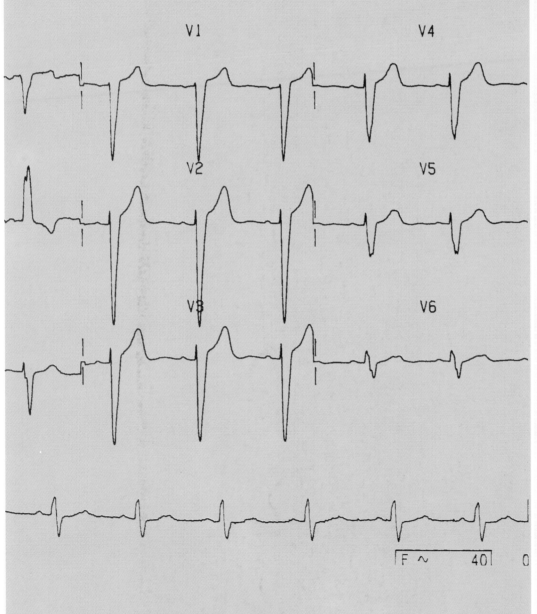

CASE 28

A 75-year-old lady with pneumonia

Right bundle branch block (RBBB)

- QRS duration of 120 ms (3 small squares) or more.
- Secondary R wave (R') in lead V1.

- Other features:
  - slurring of S wave in the lateral leads V4–6, I and aVL
  - the T wave tends to be opposite to the terminal QRS component, i.e. T wave inversion in the septal leads (V1–3) may be seen.

FEATURES OF THIS ECG

- Sinus tachycardia, 114 b.p.m., normal QRS axis
- Diagnostic features of RBBB (Fig. 28.1):
  - broad QRS, 145 ms
  - secondary R wave in V1, rSR' pattern
- Other features of RBBB:
  - T wave inversion (Fig. 28.1)
  - slurred S wave (Fig. 28.2)
- Terminal negative component of P wave in lead V1 (Fig. 28.1)
  - possible left atrial abnormality

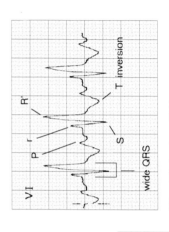

Fig. 28.1 Lead V1.

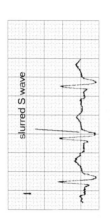

Fig. 28.2 Lead I.

Causes of right bundle branch block

↑ May occur in the absence of heart disease
↑ Fibrotic degeneration
↑ Ischaemic heart disease
↑ Hypertension
↑ Cardiomyopathy
↑ Congenital heart disease
  – atrial septal defect
  – Fallot's tetralogy
↑ Cardiomyopathy
↑ Acute, massive, pulmonary embolus

CASE 29

A healthy 29-year-old man

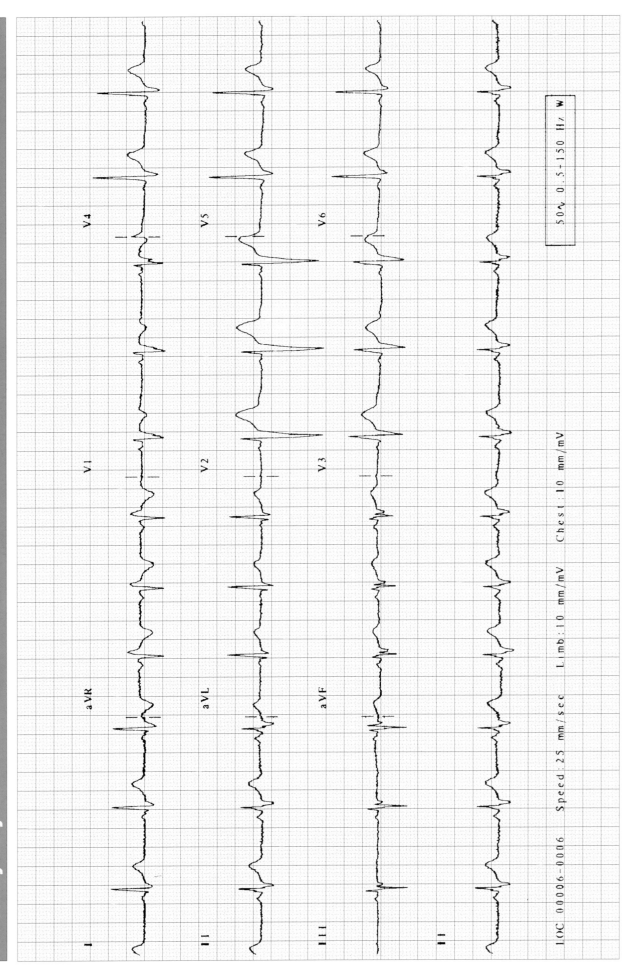

aVR   V1   V4

aVL   V2   V5

aVF   V3   V6

I

II

III

II

II

IOC 00006-0006   Speed:25 mm/sec   Limb:10 mm/mV   Chest:10 mm/mV

50〜 0.5-150 Hz W

Incomplete right bundle branch block

• QRS duration of less than 120 ms (3 small squares)

• With greater degrees of RBBB the following features appear in leads V1–2
  – decrease in depth of S wave
  – notch in upstroke of S wave
  – small r′ wave develops from this notch
  – rSr′ complex appears.

FEATURES OF THIS ECG

• Sinus arrhythmia, 66 b.p.m., leftward but normal QRS axis
• The QRS duration is about 100 ms (2.5 small squares)
• There is notching of the upstroke of the S wave in V1 (Fig. 29.1)

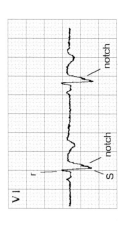

Fig. 29.1 Notched S waves.

CASE 30

An 85-year-old man with left ventricular failure

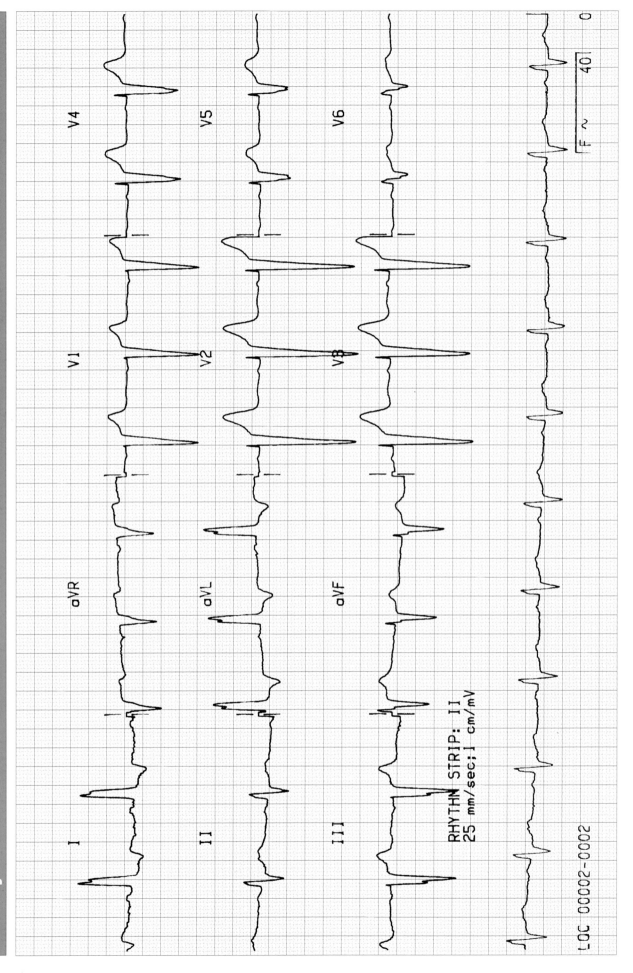

I

aVR

V1

V4

II

aVL

V2

V5

III

aVF

V3

V6

RHYTHM STRIP: II
25 mm/sec: 1 cm/mV

LOC 00002-0002

Left bundle branch block (LBBB)

- QRS duration of 120 ms (3 small squares) or more.
- No secondary R wave in lead V1.
- No Q waves in the lateral leads (V5–6, I and aVL).

- Secondary ST–T changes:
  - ST segment changes, opposite to the dominant (terminal) QRS component
  - T wave changes in the same direction as the ST segments.

These changes can mask the primary changes of acute myocardial infarction.

LBBB itself does not cause a change of QRS axis. LBBB with left axis deviation implies more extensive conduction system disease involving the main bundle proximally and the left anterior fascicle distally. It therefore carries a poorer long-term prognosis.

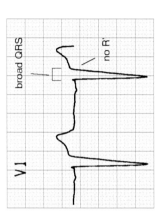

V1

broad QRS

no R'

Fig. 30.1 Lead V1.

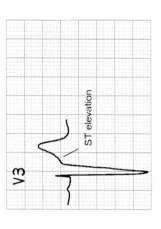

V3

ST elevation

Fig. 30.2 Secondary ST elevation.

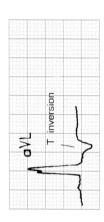

aVL

T inversion

Fig. 30.3 Secondary T wave inversion.

FEATURES OF THIS ECG

- Sinus rhythm, 66 b.p.m.
- Diagnostic features of LBBB (Fig. 30.1):
  - broad QRS, 135 ms
  - no secondary R wave in V1
  - no Q waves in the lateral leads
- Other features of LBBB:
  - ST elevation in leads V1–V4 (Fig. 30.2)
  - T wave inversion leads I and aVL (Fig. 30.3)
- Left axis deviation –30°

Causes of LBBB, left anterior or posterior hemiblock

- ↑ Ischaemic heart disease
- ↑ Hypertension
- ↑ Fibrotic degeneration
- ↑ Calcific aortic stenosis
- ↑ Congestive or hypertrophic cardiomyopathy
- ↑ Congenital heart disease
- ↑ Following cardiac surgery

CASE 31

A 56-year-old man with mitral valve disease

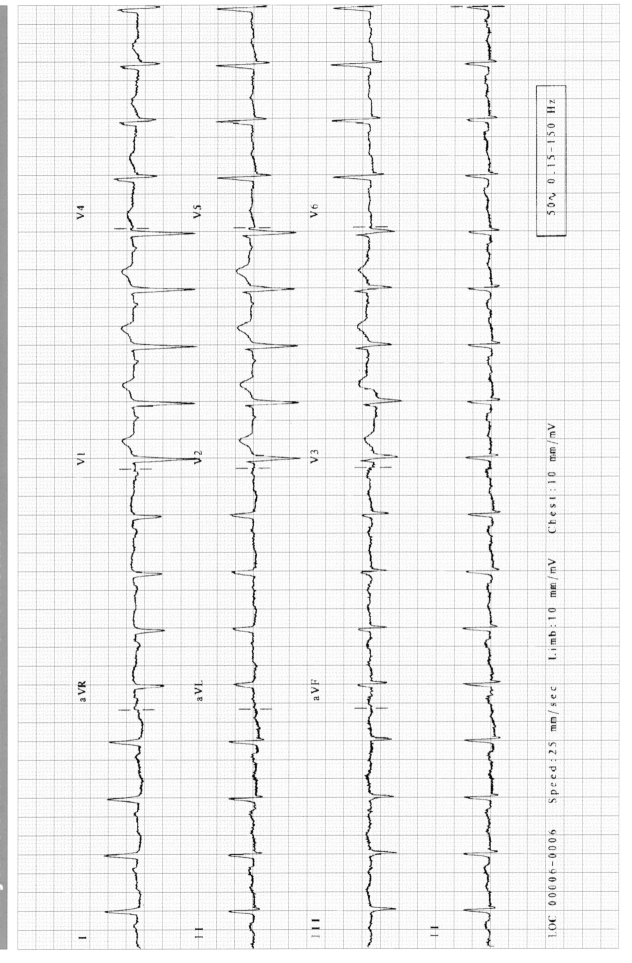

Incomplete left bundle branch block

- QRS duration of less than 120 ms (3 small squares).

- With greater degrees of LBBB the following features appear:
  - loss of small q waves in V5–6
  - notching of the R wave in leads I and aVL
  - poor R wave progression in leads V1–3
  - T wave inversion in leads V6, I and aVL
  - RsR' complexes in leads V6, I and aVL.

FEATURES OF THIS ECG

- Sinus rhythm, 100 b.p.m., normal QRS axis
- The QRS duration is about 100 ms (2.5 small squares)
- There is notching of the R wave in aVL (Fig. 31.1)
- Terminal negative component of the P wave in V1 (Fig. 31.2)
  - suggests left atrial abnormality

CLINICAL NOTE

This man had mitral regurgitation and a significantly enlarged left ventricle at echocardiography.

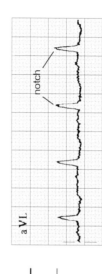

Fig. 31.1 Lead aVL.

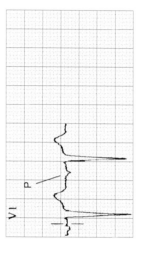

Fig. 31.2 Lead V1.

CASE 32

A 48-year-old man with ulcerative colitis, preoperative recording

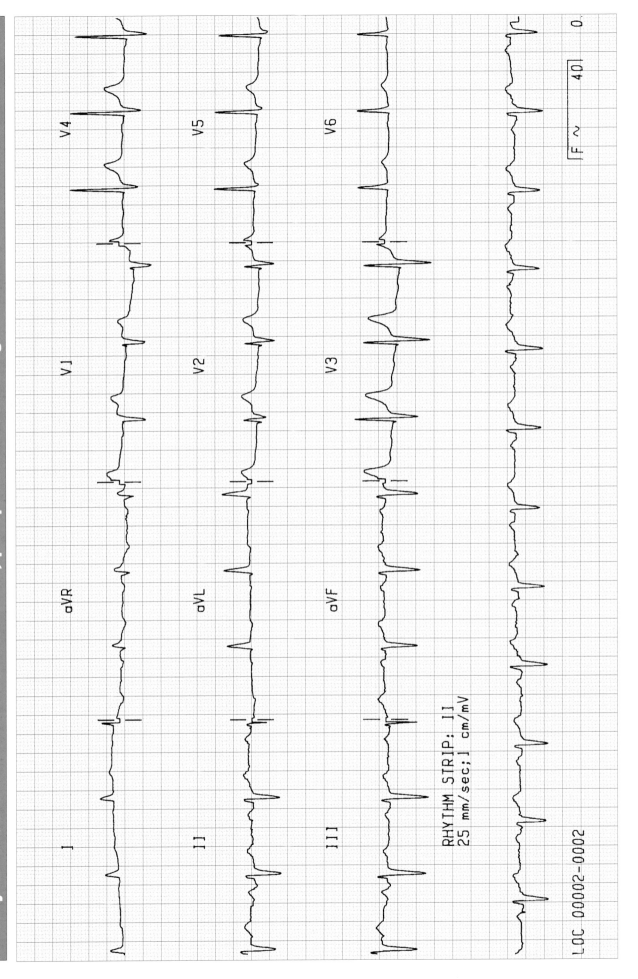

I

aVR

V1

V4

II

aVL

V2

V5

III

aVF

V3

V6

RHYTHM STRIP: II
25 mm/sec; 1 cm/mV

LOC 00002-0002

F ~   40

Left anterior hemiblock

- Axis more negative than −30°.
- Initial r wave in all the inferior leads (II, III and aVF).
- Absence of other causes of left axis deviation.

Other features:
– prominent q wave in I and aVL
– slurred terminal r wave in aVR and aVL
– loss of initial q wave in leads V5 and V6
– flat or inverted T in I and aVL.

FEATURES OF THIS ECG

- Sinus rhythm, 72 b.p.m.
- Diagnostic features of left anterior hemiblock:
  – axis approximately −60° (Fig. 32.1)
  – initial r wave in the inferior leads (Fig. 32.2)

- Other features of left anterior hemiblock:
  – slurred terminal r wave in aVR
  – absent q waves in V5 and V6
  – T wave inversion in aVL (Fig. 32.3)

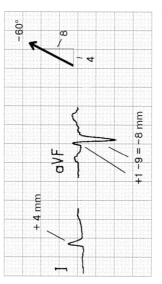

Fig. 32.1 Left axis deviation.

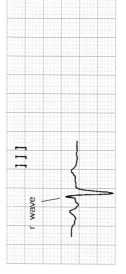

Fig. 32.2 Initial r wave.

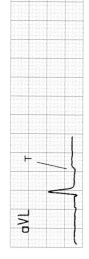

Fig. 32.3 T wave inversion.

Causes of left axis deviation

↑ Left anterior hemiblock
↑ Left ventricular hypertrophy (but not more negative than −30°)
↑ Wolff–Parkinson–White syndrome
↑ Q waves of inferior myocardial infarction
↑ Hyperkalaemia
↑ Tricuspid atresia
↑ Ostium primum ASD
↑ Artificial cardiac pacing
↑ Emphysema
↑ Injection of contrast into left coronary artery

A 63-year-old man with left ventricular failure

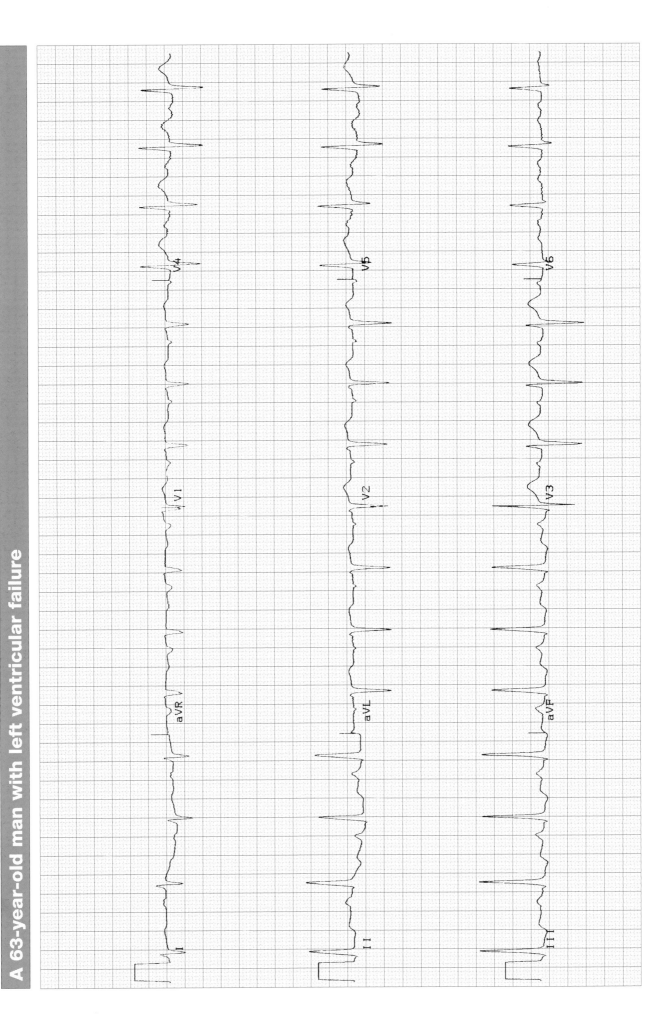

Left posterior hemiblock

Left posterior hemiblock cannot be proven on an isolated 12-lead ECG. An old recording and clinical information are needed to make a diagnosis. It is usually seen in combination with significant left ventricular disease.

- Axis between 90 and 120°.
- Initial negative vector in the inferior leads (II, III and aVF).
- Absence of other causes of right axis deviation.

- Other features:
  - slight widening of the QRS
  - secondary T wave changes (inversion) in the inferior leads.

Left posterior hemiblock can form an 'S1 Q3 T3' pattern but is usually distinguished from acute pulmonary embolism, on the ECG, by large rather than small complexes (see p. 157).

FEATURES OF THIS ECG

- Sinus rhythm, 90 b.p.m.

- Features suggesting left posterior hemiblock:
  - right axis deviation +110° (Fig. 33.1)
  - initial negative vector (q wave) in leads II, III and aVF (Fig. 33. 2)
  - T wave inversion in the inferior leads
- Evidence of incomplete left bundle branch block:
  - absent small q waves in leads V5–6
  - slightly broad QRS complexes
- Negative P wave in lead V1 suggesting left atrial abnormality
  - the combination of left atrial abnormality and large voltage deflections would suggest left ventricular hypertrophy

CLINICAL NOTE

This man had no clinical or echocardiographic evidence of right ventricular hypertrophy. He did not have a history of inferior MI or chronic lung disease.

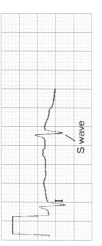

Fig. 33.1   Lead I negative.

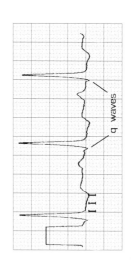

Fig. 33.2   Lead III.

Causes of right axis deviation

↑ Left posterior hemiblock
↑ Normal finding in children and tall thin adults
↑ Right ventricular hypertrophy
↑ Chronic lung disease even without pulmonary hypertension
↑ Significant left ventricular disease
↑ Anterolateral myocardial infarction
↑ Pulmonary embolus
↑ Atrial septal defect
↑ Ventricular septal defect

CASE 34

A 70-year-old lady with a stroke

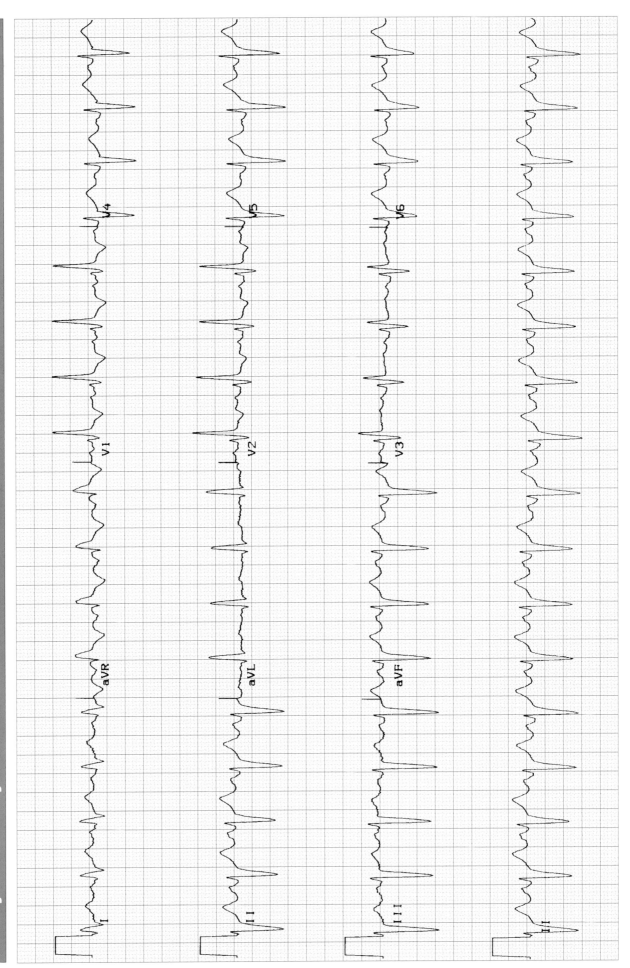

Right bundle branch block with left anterior hemiblock (bifascicular block)

- QRS duration of 120 ms (3 small squares) or more.
- A secondary R wave (R') in lead V1.
- Axis more negative than −30°.
- Initial r wave in all the inferior leads (II, III and aVF).
- Absence of other causes of left axis deviation.

FEATURES OF THIS ECG

- Sinus tachycardia, 108 b.p.m.
- Features of RBBB:
  - QRS duration approximately 140 ms and rsR' in V1 (Fig. 34.1)
  - T wave inversion in V1 and V2 (Fig. 34.1)
- Features of left anterior hemiblock:
  - abnormal left axis deviation −80° (Fig. 34.2)
  - initial r wave in the inferior leads (Fig. 34.3)
- Terminal negative component of P wave in lead V1 (Fig. 34.1)
  - suggesting left atrial abnormality

CLINICAL NOTE

This was a coincidental finding in this lady.

The combination of RBBB and left posterior hemiblock is also a 'bifascicular block' and is said to be more likely to progress to complete heart block.

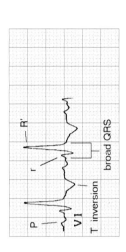

Fig. 34.1 Features of RBBB.

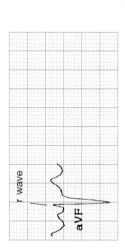

Fig. 34.2 Left axis deviation.

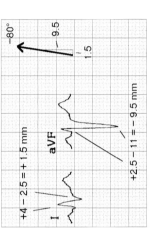

Fig. 34.3 Inferior lead.

CASE 35

A 74-year-old lady referred to hospital with a wide complex tachycardia

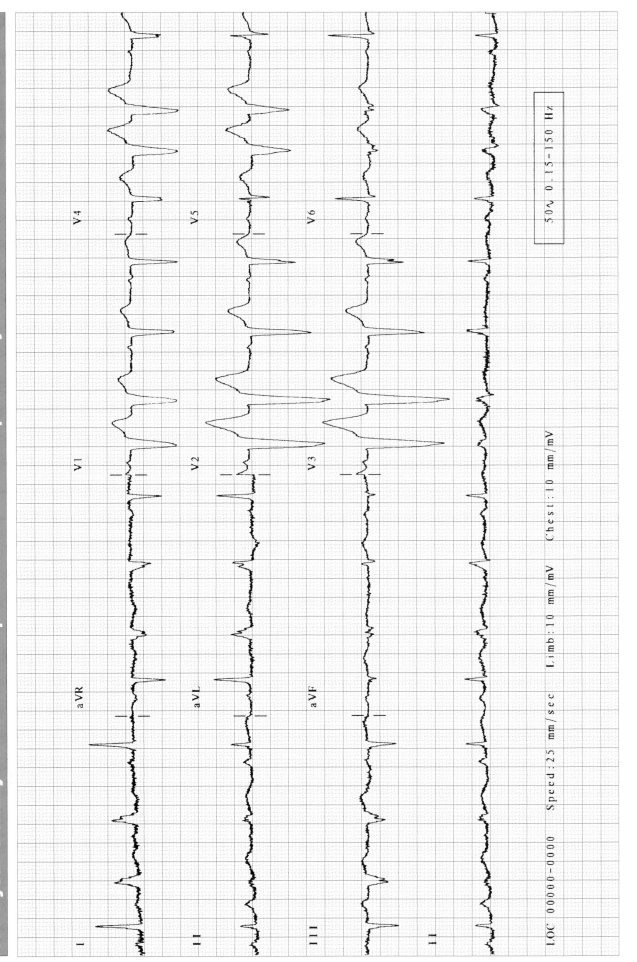

LOC 00000-0000   Speed:25 mm/sec   Limb:10 mm/mV   Chest:10 mm/mV

50~ 0.15-150 Hz

Phasic aberrant ventricular conduction

- Sometimes the degree of bundle branch block depends on the timing; shorter R–R intervals producing more aberrant conduction.

CLINICAL NOTE

The ambulance ECG strips showed atrial flutter with complete left bundle branch block pattern.

FEATURES OF THIS ECG

- Sinus rhythm with frequent atrial premature beats
- Rate variable 75–130 b.p.m., normal QRS axis

The recording represents a 10-second period of time from left to right. The complexes in the rhythm strip coincide with those in the leads above which helps identify abnormalities.

- Phasic aberrant ventricular conduction (Fig. 35.1):
  - complexes 1, 2, 4 and 5 are supraventricular
  - each one is preceded by a P wave
  - complex 3 is indeterminate
  - shorter R–R intervals are associated with broader QRS complexes
- Phasic aberrant conduction is also suggested elsewhere (Fig. 35.2)

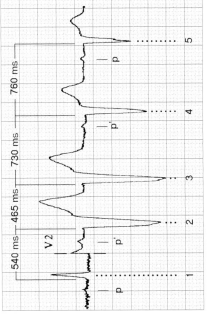

Fig. 35.1   Lead V2.

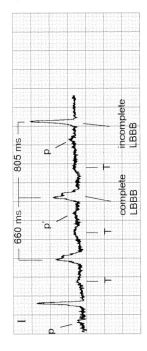

Fig. 35.2   Lead I.

Causes of 'aberrant' conduction

→ Permanent:
  - bundle branch block
  - ventricular pre-excitation
→ Rate related:
  - acceleration-dependent aberrancy (shown here)
  - deceleration-dependent aberrancy

HEART BLOCK

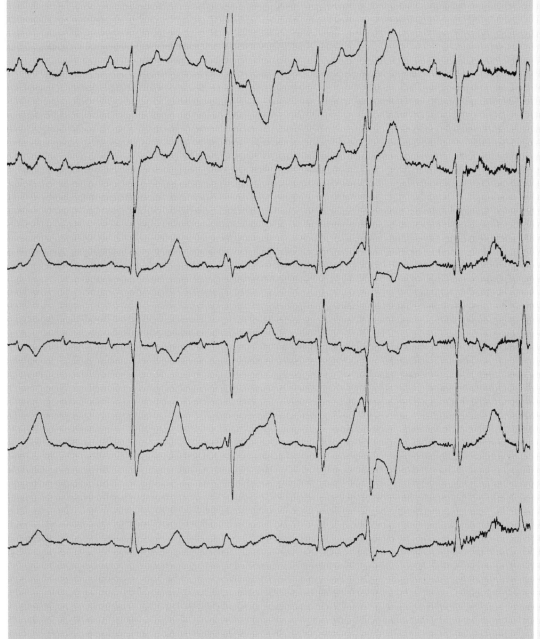

A 78-year-old man with diabetes

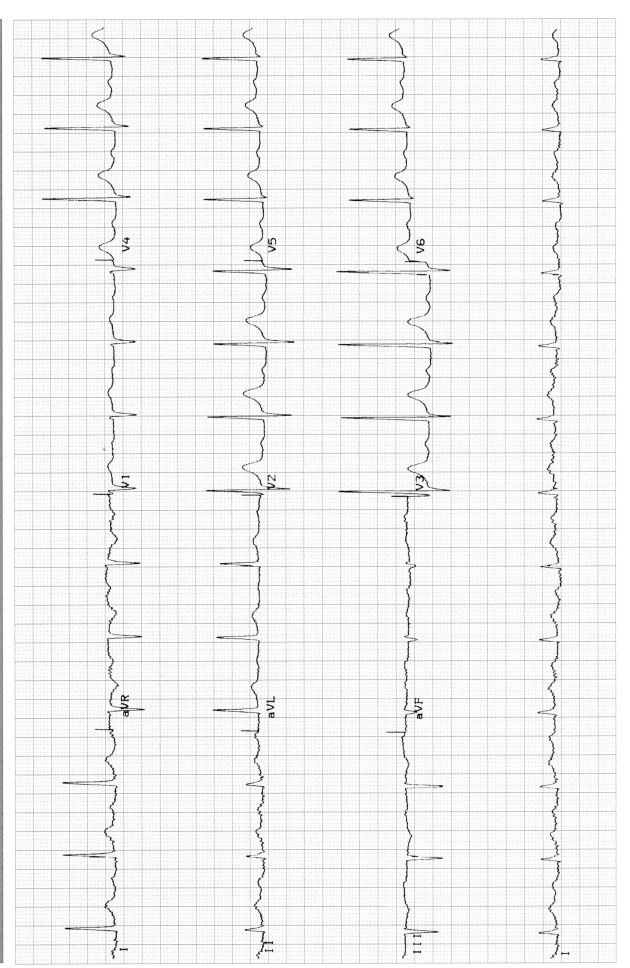

First degree heart block

- A PR interval of greater than 200 ms (5 small squares). In practice a PR interval of 200–220 ms is of dubious clinical significance.

FEATURES OF THIS ECG

- Sinus rhythm, 75 b.p.m., normal QRS axis
- Features of first degree heart block
  – long PR interval, 320 ms (Fig. 36.1)
- Probable old posteroinferior myocardial infarction

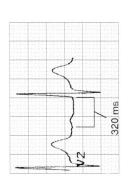

320 ms

Fig. 36.1 Long PR interval.

Common causes of a long PR interval

- ↑ Increased vagal tone
- ↑ Idiopathic
- ↑ Ischaemic heart disease
- ↑ Rheumatic carditis
- ↑ Digoxin toxicity
- ↑ Electrolyte disturbances

CASE 37

A 48-year-old man with 2 days of chest pain

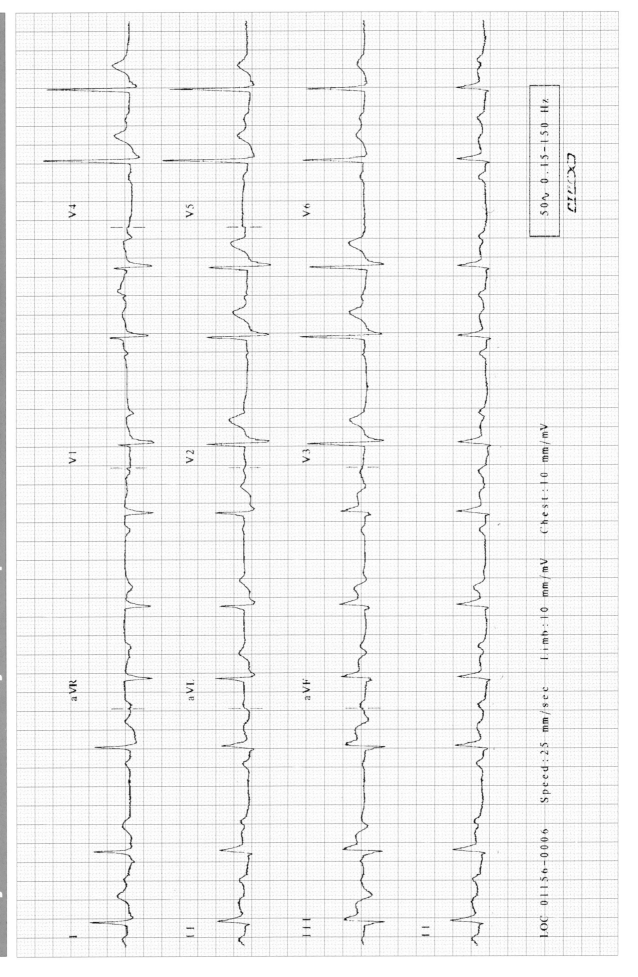

aVR   V1   V4

aVL   V2   V5

aVF   V3   V6

I

II

III

II

LOC 01156-0006   Speed:25 mm/sec   Limb:10 mm/mV   Chest:10 mm/mV

50s 0.15-150 Hz

Second degree heart block – Mobitz type 1 or Wenckebach AV block

- The PR interval becomes progressively longer until a P wave is not conducted. The pause that follows failed conduction is less than fully compensatory (i.e. less than two normal sinus intervals).

FEATURES OF THIS ECG

- Second degree heart block (3:2 and 4:3 AV conduction):
  - constant atrial rate of 96 b.p.m.
  - average ventricular rate of 66 b.p.m.
- Normal QRS axis
- Features of Wenckebach AV block:
  - progressive lengthening of the PR interval followed by failure of AV conduction (Fig. 37.1)
- Features of acute inferior myocardial infarction (Fig. 37.2):
  - ST elevation
  - Q waves

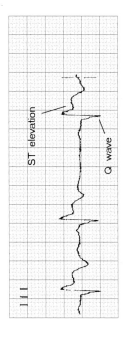

Fig. 37.1 Rhythm strip.

Fig. 37.2 Lead III.

CLINICAL NOTE

This man had an acute inferior MI with transient second degree heart block. He did not require pacing. Wenckebach block can progress to complete heart block; however, the escape rhythm usually arises in the proximal His bundle (narrow QRS) and is well tolerated.

Common causes of Wenckebach AV block

- ↑ Inferior myocardial infarction
- ↑ Drug intoxication (digoxin, beta blockers, calcium antagonists)
- ↑ Heightened vagal tone (e.g. athlete)

CASE 38

An 86-year-old lady with episodes of syncope

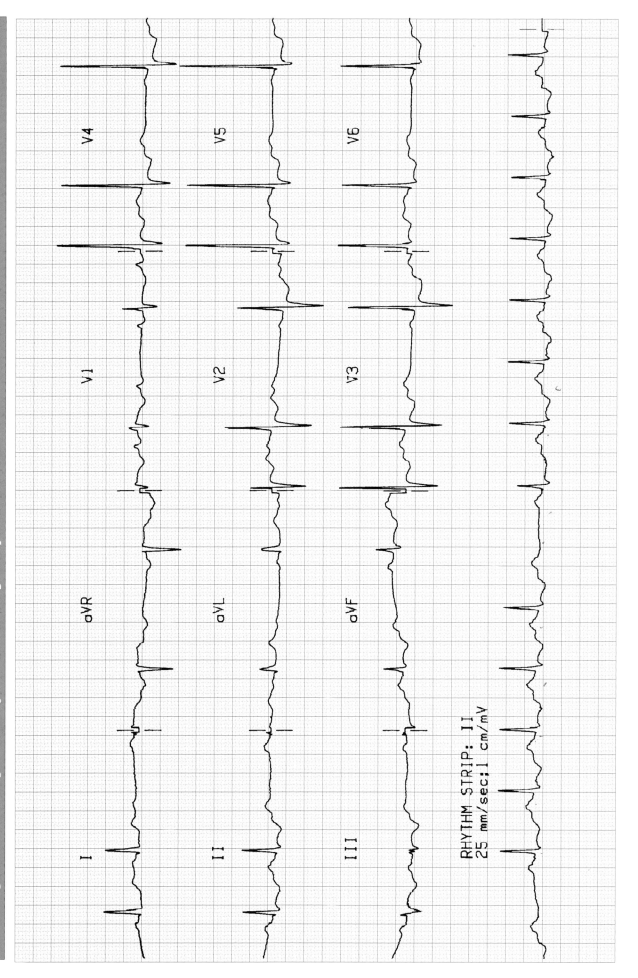

I

aVR

V1

V4

II

aVL

V2

V5

III

aVF

V3

V6

RHYTHM STRIP: II
25 mm/sec;1 cm/mV

Second degree heart block – Mobitz type 2

- Most beats are conducted with a constant PR interval. Occasionally there is an atrial contraction without a subsequent ventricular contraction, i.e. there is intermittent blocking of conduction either through the AV node or, more commonly, the His–Purkinje system. Disease of the His–Purkinje system is most often associated with a prolonged QRS duration.

FEATURES OF THIS ECG

- Sinus rhythm, 90 b.p.m., normal QRS axis
- Features of Mobitz type 2 AV block (Fig. 38.1):
  – the PR interval is constant
  – the first and seventh P waves on the rhythm strip are not followed by a QRS complex
- Features of left ventricular hypertrophy:
  – SV2 + RV5 > 35 mm
  – widespread ST depression and T wave inversion

CLINICAL NOTE

This lady had a permanent pacemaker inserted. Unlike Wenckebach block, Mobitz type 2 block is usually due to disease of the His bundle rather than the AV node and if it progresses to CHB the escape rhythm tends to be slow with wide QRS complexes.

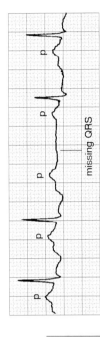

Fig. 38.1 Rhythm strip.

Common causes of Mobitz type 2 AV block

↑ Degenerative disease of the conducting system
↑ Anteroseptal infarction

CASE 39

A 70-year-old man with bradycardia following cardiac surgery

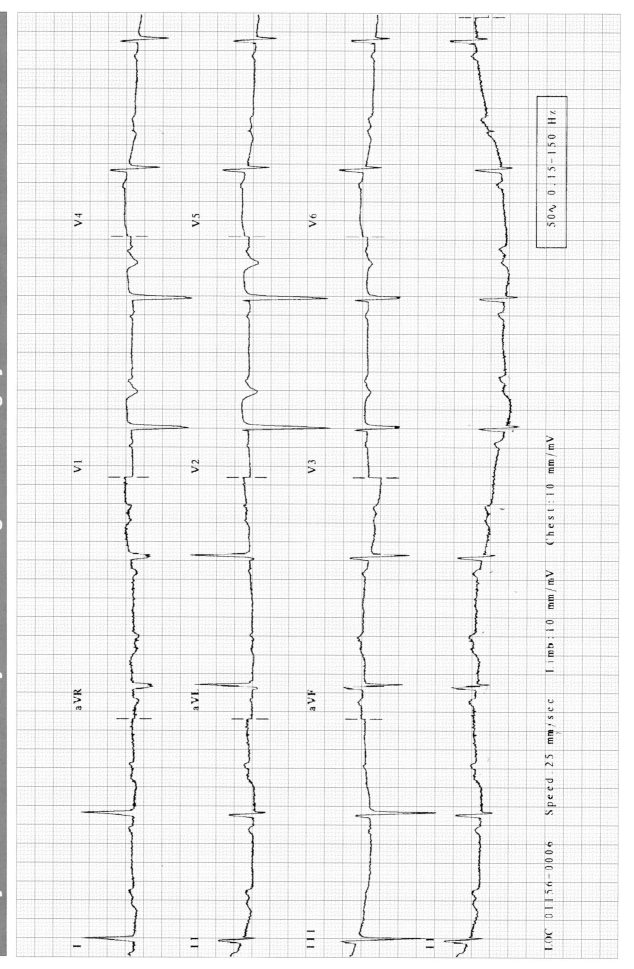

LOC 01156-0006   Speed 25 mm/sec   Limb:10 mm/mV   Chest:10 mm/mV

50∿ 0.15-150 Hz

Second degree heart block – 2:1 AV block

- Every second P wave is conducted to the ventricles.
- The conducted beats have a constant PR interval.

FEATURES OF THIS ECG

- Second degree heart block:
  – atrial rate 84 b.p.m.
  – ventricular rate 42 b.p.m.
- Normal QRS axis
- Narrow QRS complexes (indicating block at the level of the AV node)
- Features of 2:1 AV block:
  – alternate P waves are conducted to the ventricles (Fig. 39.1)
- Features of left ventricular hypertrophy:
  – R aVL > 11 mm

CLINICAL NOTE

This man recently underwent aortic valve replacement for critical aortic stenosis. He subsequently developed complete heart block and required a permanent pacemaker. Presumably his AV node was damaged during the surgery.

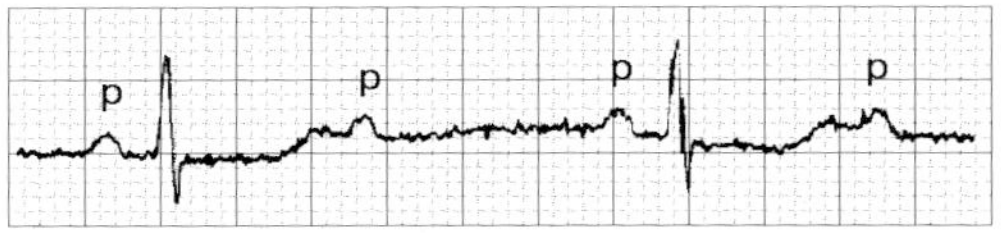

Fig. 39.1   Rhythm strip.

CASE 40

A 54-year-old man with poor exercise tolerance

Second degree heart block – high grade

- The atrioventricular conduction ratio is 3:1 or higher.
- The PR interval of conducted atrial impulses is constant.

FEATURES OF THIS ECG

- Second degree heart block:
  - atrial rate 120 b.p.m.
  - ventricular rate 40 b.p.m.
- Features of high grade AV block:
  - constant PR interval of conducted atrial beats (long PR, 240 ms)
  - There are three P waves for each QRS complex (Fig. 40.1); this is 3:1 block
- Two ventricular premature beats (Fig. 40.2)
- Features of bifascicular block (RBBB + left anterior hemiblock):
  - prolonged QRS duration, 160 ms
  - a secondary R wave in V1
  - left axis deviation
  - initial r wave in the inferior leads
- Evidence of possible previous anterior myocardial infarction:
  - Q waves in the anterolateral leads (Fig. 40.3)

CLINICAL NOTE

This ECG was taken during an outpatient exercise tolerance test. This man had suffered an anterior myocardial infarction 6 weeks previously and complained of poor exercise tolerance and dizzy spells. The above conduction abnormalities developed after 4 minutes on the treadmill. He was fitted with a permanent pacemaker.

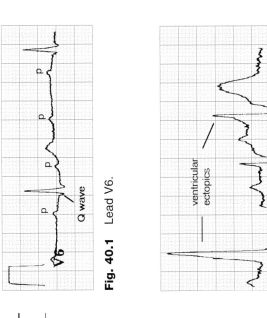

Fig. 40.1   Lead V6.

Fig. 40.2   Lead aVF.

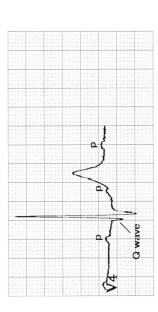

Fig. 40.3   Lead V4.

CASE 41

An 84-year-old man presenting with 'collapse'

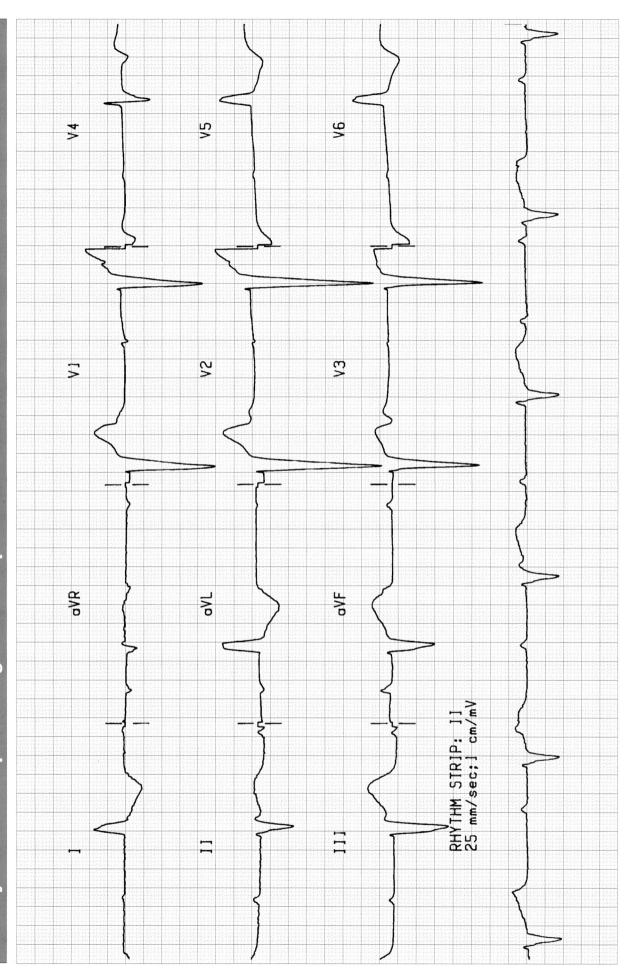

I

aVR

V1

V4

II

aVL

V2

V5

III

aVF

V3

V6

RHYTHM STRIP: II
25 mm/sec; 1 cm/mV

Third degree heart block – wide complex escape

● Atrial contraction is normal but no beats are conducted to the ventricles, i.e. there is complete AV dissociation.

When the AV block occurs in the lower parts of the His–Purkinje system the ventricular escape complexes have wide QRS morphology. Third degree heart block is also known as complete heart block.

FEATURES OF THIS ECG

● Complete heart block:
  – atrial rate 70 b.p.m.
  – ventricular rate 31 b.p.m.
● Features of complete heart block:
  – normal atrial contraction with failure to conduct to the ventricles (Fig. 41.1)
  – wide complex idioventricular escape rhythm with LBBB pattern

CLINICAL NOTE

This man's complete heart block was thought to be on the basis of degenerative disease of the infranodal conducting system. He was fitted with a permanent pacemaker.

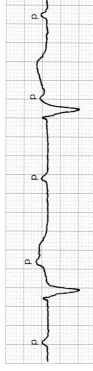

Fig. 41.1 Rhythm strip.

Causes of third degree (complete) heart block

↑ Infranodal degenerative fibrosis
↑ Myocardial infarction
↑ Drugs – digoxin, beta blockers
↑ Congenital (rare)

A 22-year-old lady with a history of poor exercise tolerance

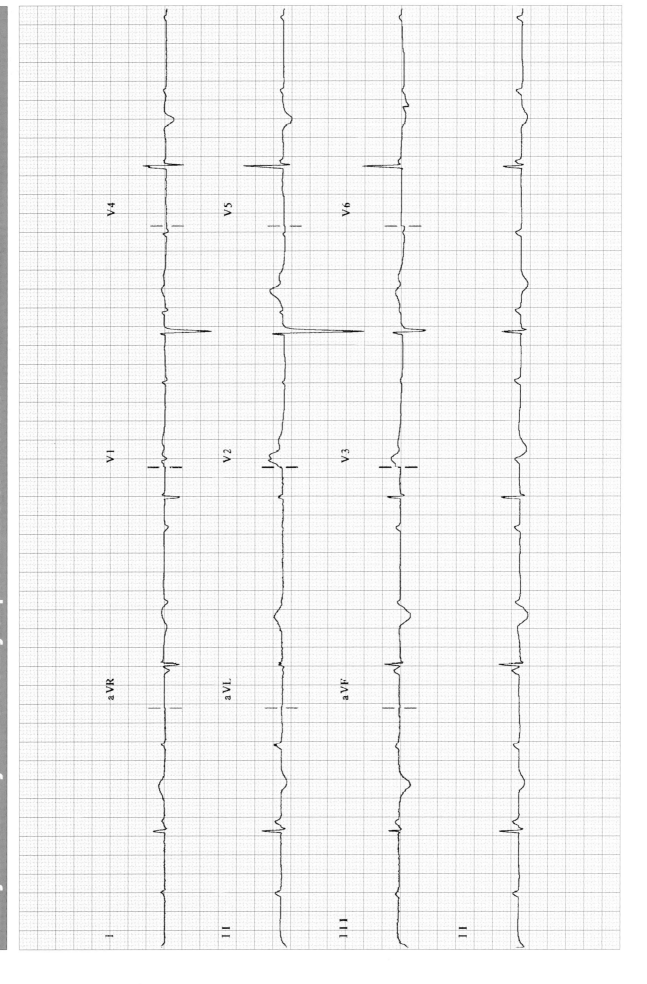

Third degree heart block – narrow complex escape

- Atrial contraction is normal but no beats are conducted to the ventricles, i.e. there is complete AV dissociation.

When the AV block is high in the His–Purkinje system the escape rhythm is classically of narrow QRS morphology.

FEATURES OF THIS ECG

- Complete heart block:
  - atrial rate 75 b.p.m.
  - ventricular rate 34 b.p.m.
- Features of complete heart block:
  - P waves completely dissociated from the QRS complexes (Fig. 42.1)
  - the escape rhythm is narrow complex indicating that the ventricular pacemaker is high in the His–Purkinje system

CLINICAL NOTE

This lady had congenital complete heart block. The ECG was taken when her pacing system became infected and had to be removed. Congenital complete heart block is typically localised to the AV node producing narrow QRS escape complexes.

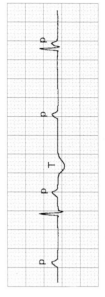

Fig. 42.1   Rhythm strip.

CASE 43

An 84-year-old lady with dizziness and poor mobility

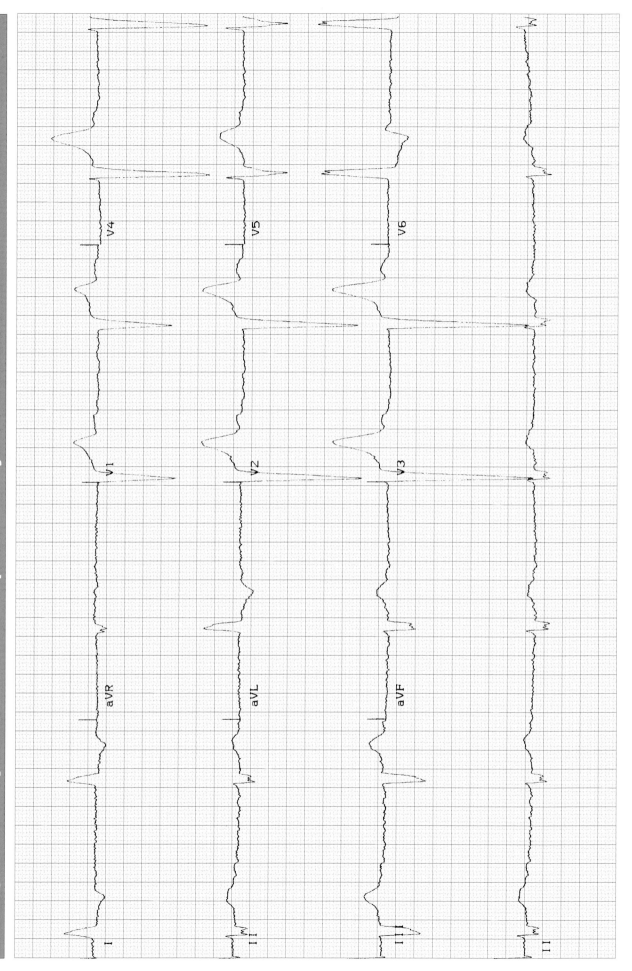

Third degree heart block and atrial fibrillation

- There are no P waves.
- Fibrillary waves of irregular atrial activation may be seen.
- In contrast to atrial fibrillation with normal AV conduction there is a regular, slow ventricular escape rhythm which may display narrow or wide QRS morphology depending on the location of the escape pacemaker.

FEATURES OF THIS ECG

- Atrial fibrillation:
  - there are no P waves
  - there are prominent fibrillary waves (Fig. 43.1)
- Complete heart block:
  - ventricular rate 38 b.p.m.
  - wide complex idioventricular escape rhythm with LBBB block pattern

CLINICAL NOTE

This lady had longstanding atrial fibrillation and was not taking digoxin. A permanent ventricular pacemaker was implanted and her mobility improved allowing her to live independently.

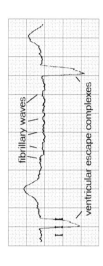

Fig. 43.1 Lead III.

PACEMAKERS

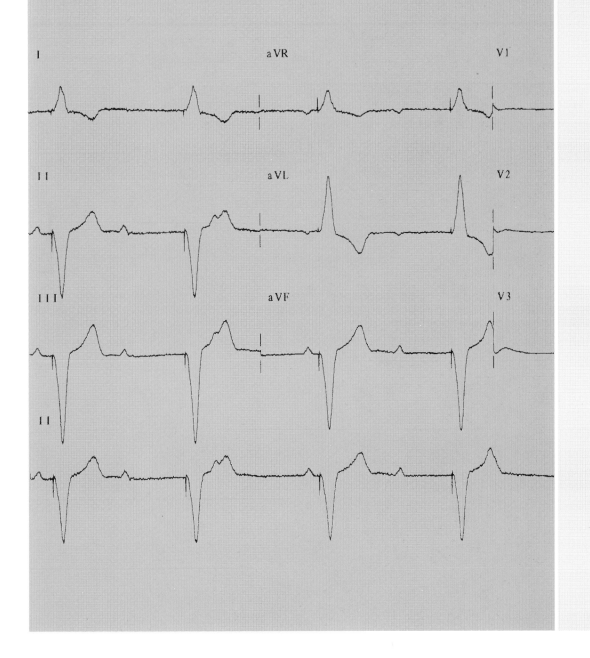

An 82-year-old man who had presented with collapse

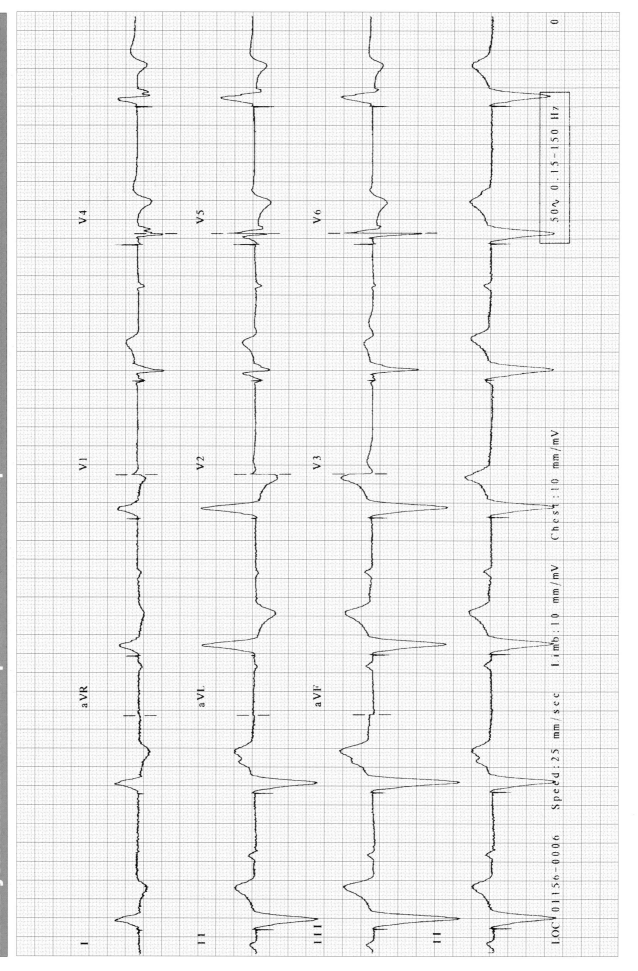

Ventricular pacemaker

- There is a pacing spike before the QRS complex.
- The paced complexes are wide and of abnormal morphology (usually resembles LBBB as the tip of the pacing wire is most commonly placed at the apex of the right ventricle).

FEATURES OF THIS ECG

- Paced rhythm, ventricular rate 42 b.p.m.
  – atrial rate 66 b.p.m., AV dissociation is present
- There are pacing spikes before each QRS complex (Fig. 44.1)
- An occasional pacing spike is obscured by a P wave (Fig. 44.2)
- Abnormal QRS complexes with a LBBB pattern

CLINICAL NOTE

This was a patient with a temporary pacing wire inserted for symptomatic complete heart block (CHB). He needed permanent pacing. This ECG was taken when the paced rate was slowed to allow assessment of the underlying rhythm which has remained as CHB.

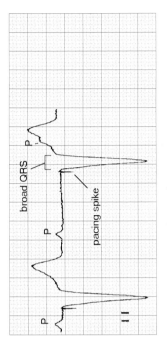

Fig. 44.1 Ventricular pacing.

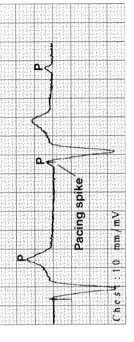

Fig. 44.2 Rhythm strip.

Pacemaker nomenclature

Chamber(s) paced	Chamber(s) sensed	Response to sensing	Programmability
A = atrium	A = atrium	T = triggered	P = simple programmable
V = ventricle	V = ventricle	I = inhibited	M = multiprogrammable
D = dual (A+V)	D = dual (A+V)	D = dual (T+I)	C = communicating
O = none	O = none	O = no sensing	R = rate modulation

Example: VVIR pacemaker – paces the ventricle, senses the ventricle, is inhibited by sensed spontaneous ventricular activity and has rate modulation.

CASE 45

A 60-year-old lady with a history of blackouts

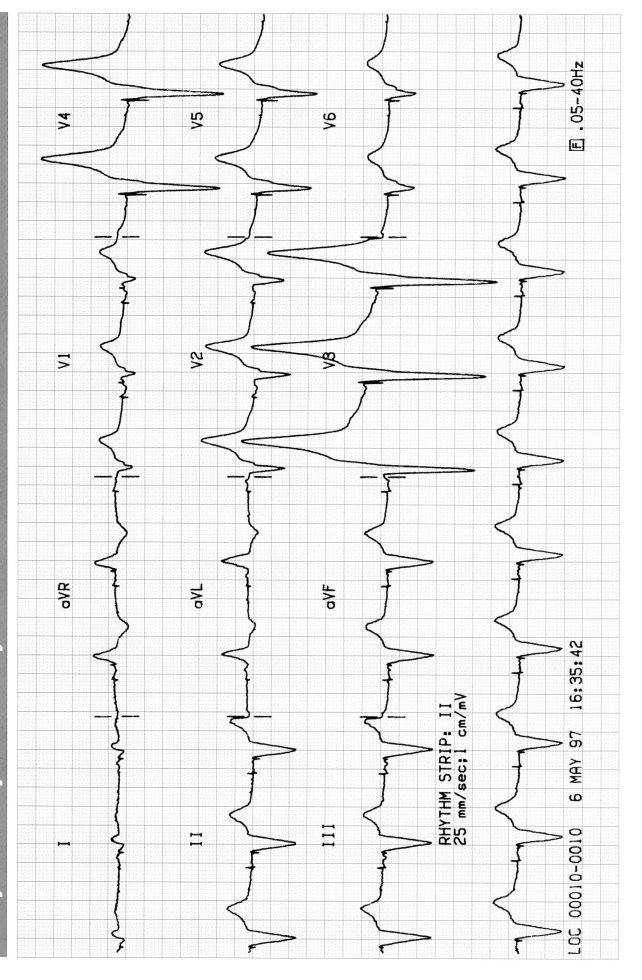

I

aVR

V1

V4

II

aVL

V2

V5

III

aVF

V3

V6

RHYTHM STRIP: II
25 mm/sec; 1 cm/mV

LOC 00010-0010   6 MAY 97   16:35:42   .05-40Hz

Dual chamber pacing (AV sequential pacing)

- Pacing spikes may precede the P wave and/or the QRS complex.

Modern dual chamber pacemakers such as DDD models sense intrinsic atrial and ventricular activity and only pace the appropriate chambers as required. The morphology of the induced P wave may be abnormal or closely resemble the normal P wave depending on the position of the pacing electrode in the right atrium. The morphology of the induced QRS also depends on the position of the ventricular wire but usually resembles a LBBB pattern.

FEATURES OF THIS ECG

- Dual chamber paced rhythm, 60 b.p.m.
- Pacing spikes preceding each P wave and QRS complex (Fig. 45.1)

CLINICAL NOTE

This lady had a permanent pacemaker inserted for sick sinus syndrome.

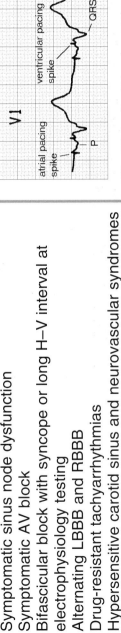

Fig. 45.1 Dual chamber pacing.

Common indications for pacemaker insertion

↑ ↑ Symptomatic sinus node dysfunction
↑ Symptomatic AV block
↑ Bifascicular block with syncope or long H–V interval at electrophysiology testing
↑ Alternating LBBB and RBBB
↑ Drug-resistant tachyarrhythmias
↑ Hypersensitive carotid sinus and neurovascular syndromes

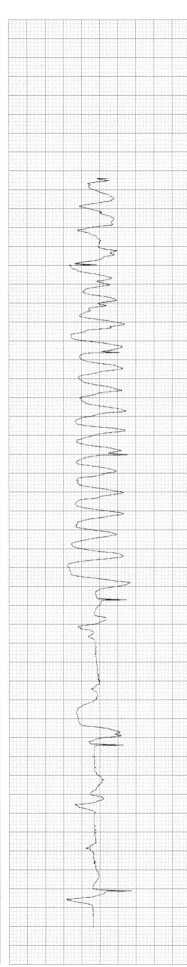

CASE 46

A 58-year-old man with complete heart block after an anterior MI

Problems with pacemakers – failure to sense

• Pacemaker firing despite the presence of spontaneous myocardial depolarisation may be hazardous as shown here.

FEATURES OF THIS ECG

• The pacemaker has discharged whilst the ventricle is repolarising (T wave) causing ventricular tachycardia (Fig. 46.1)

CLINICAL NOTE

This man had a temporary pacing wire that had stopped sensing because of damage to the wire near entry to the skin. It needed to be replaced.

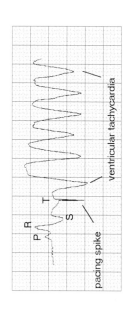

Fig. 46.1   Failure to sense.

Causes of failure to sense/capture

↑ Sensing threshold too high
↑ Critical positioning of wire tip
↑ Endocardial disease (e.g. old MI, endocarditis)
↑ Mechanical damage to wire
↑ Other equipment failure

A 79-year-old man with a recent pacemaker insertion

Problems with pacemakers – failure to capture

- Pacemaker firing but failing to pace the myocardium.

FEATURES OF THIS ECG

- Dual chamber pacemaker
- Upper rhythm strip:
  - normal 'physiological' ventricular pacing, 75 b.p.m.
  - The normal P waves are sensed and followed by paced ventricular beats (Fig. 47.1)
  - LBBB morphology of QRS complexes
- Lower rhythm strip:
  - failure of ventricular capture (Fig. 47.2) but normal ventricular sensing (Fig. 47.3)
  - slow ventricular escape rhythm, 33 b.p.m.
  - there is normal atrial pacing (Fig. 47.3); note the different shape of the paced P wave
  - return to normal pacing at the end of the strip

CLINICAL NOTE

These rhythm strips were taken from an elderly man who had recently undergone permanent pacemaker insertion. He had to return to theatre the following morning for repositioning of the ventricular pacing wire. As can be seen from the lower rhythm strip, the underlying abnormality was complete heart block.

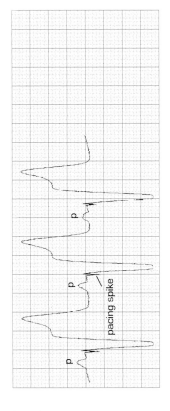

Fig. 47.1 Physiological pacing.

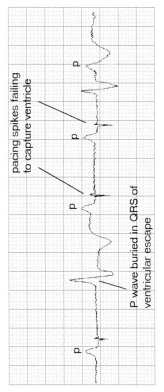

Fig. 47.2 Failure to capture.

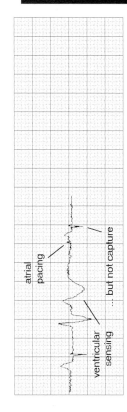

Fig. 47.3 Lower strip.

ISCHAEMIC HEART DISEASE

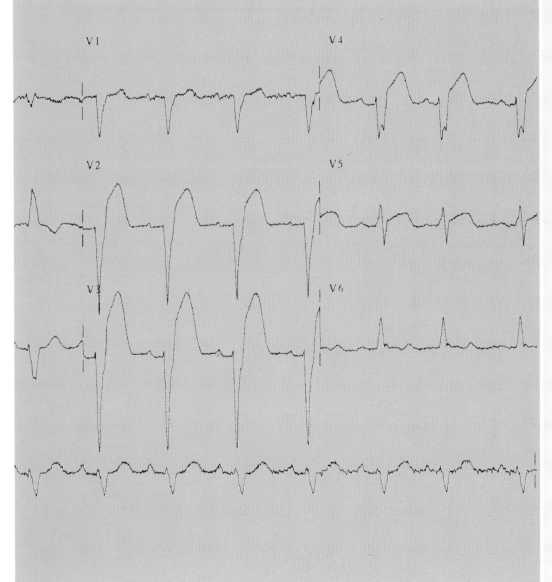

A 47-year-old man during an exercise tolerance test

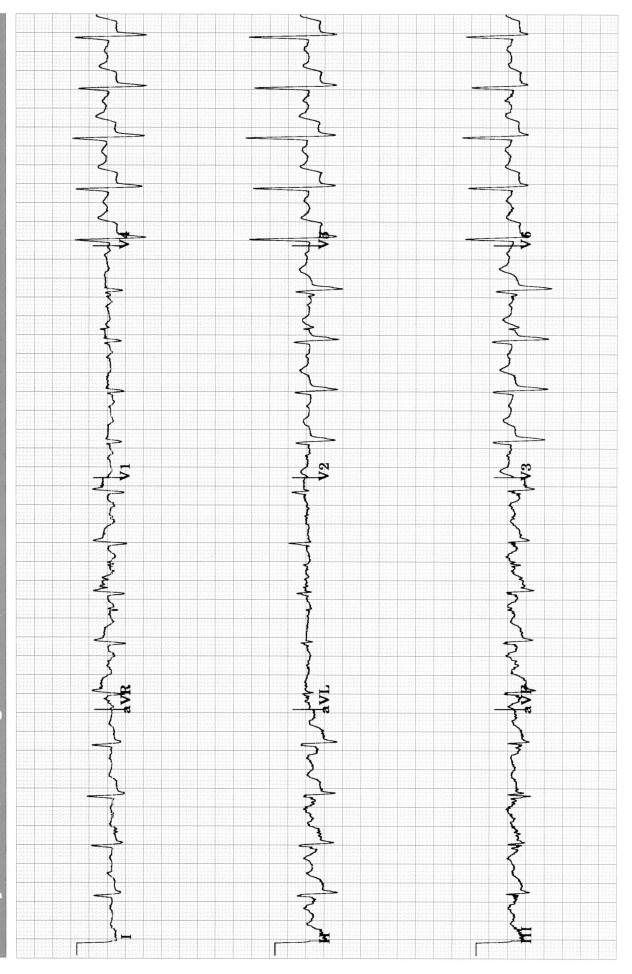

Myocardial ischaemia – ST depression

Horizontal ST depression is strongly suggestive of ischaemia in an appropriate clinical setting. Sloping ST depression is a less reliable indicator of ischaemia.

FEATURES OF THIS ECG

- Sinus tachycardia, 110 b.p.m., normal QRS axis
- Horizontal ST depression in the inferior and lateral leads (Fig. 48.1)

CLINICAL NOTE

This ECG was taken at 3 minutes 20 seconds. The patient developed chest pain and the above ECG changes.

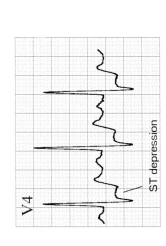

Fig. 48.1 Horizontal ST depression.

Common causes of ST depression

↑ Horizontal:
  – ischaemia
  – subendocardial infarction
  – reciprocal to ST elevation (acute injury)
↑ Sloping:
  – ventricular hypertrophy
  – digoxin
  – ischaemia
  – hyperkalaemia
  – bundle branch block

CASE 49

A 42-year-old man with chest pain

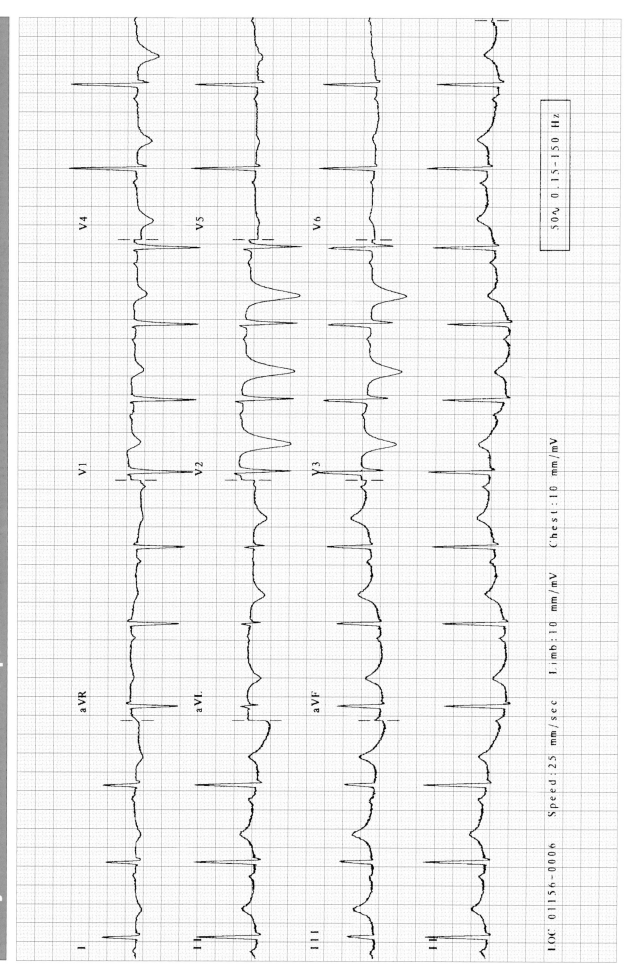

LOC: 01156-0006   Speed: 25 mm/sec   Limb: 10 mm/mV   Chest: 10 mm/mV

50~ 0.15-150 Hz

Myocardial ischaemia – T wave inversion

There are no definitive criteria for the normal T wave and numerous conditions other than ischaemia can cause T wave changes (see next page). Inversion of the T wave is considered abnormal in V3–6, I, II and aVF in most adults. T wave inversion is relatively non-specific for ischaemia unless it is deep and symmetrical ('arrowhead') inversion.

FEATURES OF THIS ECG

- Sinus rhythm, 75 b.p.m., normal QRS axis
- Deep and symmetrical T wave inversion in the anterior leads, V1–5, I and aVL (Fig. 49.1)
- Long QT interval

CLINICAL NOTE

This patient had post-infarct angina. His ECG the previous day had been normal. Subsequent angiography showed a 50% stenosis in the left anterior descending coronary artery with thrombus visible in the lumen. The ECG returned to normal with 4 days of i.v. heparin.

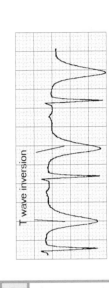

Fig. 49.1 V2, 'Arrowhead' T wave inversion.

Causes of deep symmetrical T wave inversion

↑ ↑ Subendocardial ischaemia
↑ ↑ Subendocardial infarction (non Q-wave infarction)
↑ Hypertrophic obstructive cardiomyopathy
↑ Juvenile pattern
↑ Intracranial haemorrhage

CASE 50

A 61-year-old lady – routine preoperative ECG

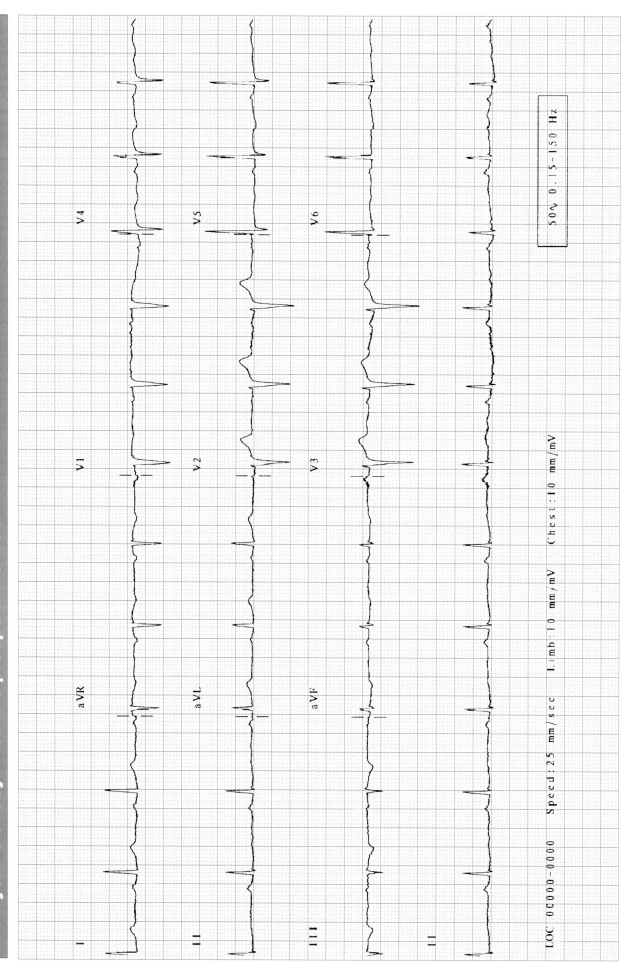

LOC 0C000-0000   Speed:25 mm/sec   Limb:10 mm/mV   Chest:10 mm/mV

50~ 0.15-150 Hz

Myocardial ischaemia – non-specific changes

Usually the ECG changes of ischaemia are more subtle than those shown in the previous two examples and are referred to as non-specific ST and T wave changes. These changes include minimal or sloping ST depression, T wave flattening, abnormally tall T waves, and minimal T wave inversion.

FEATURES OF THIS ECG

- Sinus rhythm, 72 b.p.m., normal QRS axis
- T wave flattening in the lateral leads V4–6 (Fig. 50.1)
- Flattened T wave in II, minimal T wave inversion in leads aVF and III (Fig. 50.2)

CLINICAL NOTE

This patient had a history of stable angina. This ECG was done routinely prior to hip joint replacement surgery.

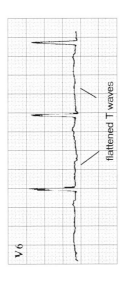

Fig. 50.1   T wave flattening.

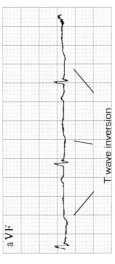

Fig. 50.2   T wave inversion.

Common causes of T wave changes

- ↑ Myocardial ischaemia
- ↑ Physiological (race, hyperventilation, anxiety, iced water)
- ↑ Left ventricular hypertrophy
- ↑ Drugs (e.g. digoxin)
- ↑ Myocarditis/pericarditis
- ↑ Pulmonary embolus
- ↑ Intraventricular conduction delay
- ↑ Electrolyte abnormalities

CASE 51

A 36-year-old man with 40 minutes of 'crushing' chest pain

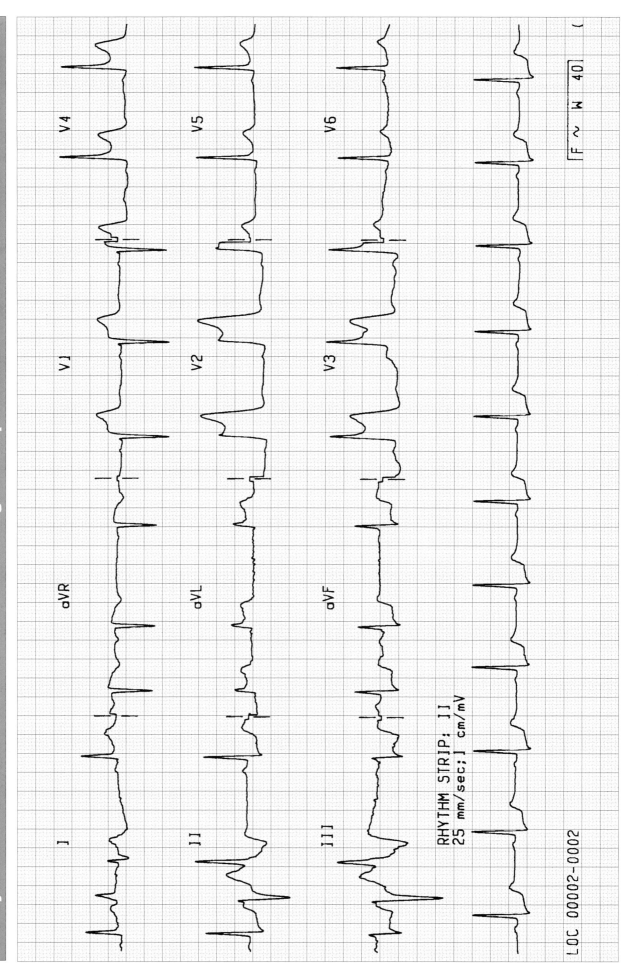

RHYTHM STRIP: II
25 mm/sec;1 cm/mV

LOC 00002-0002

Acute extensive anterior myocardial infarction

- Changes of acute injury (ST elevation) in most or all anterior leads V1–6, I and aVL.
- With or without reciprocal changes (ST depression) in the inferior leads.

(NB: Infarction can be divided into regions depending on which leads show changes; however, these should not be treated rigidly as lead positions may vary. What is important is that the pattern of acute injury is recognised and distinguished from other causes of ST elevation.)

- Reciprocal ST depression in leads II, III and aVF (Fig. 51.2) – the mirror image of the acute injury
- Two consecutive ventricular premature beats from different ectopic foci (Fig. 51.3)

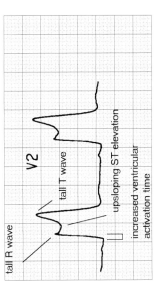

Fig. 51.1 Acute injury.

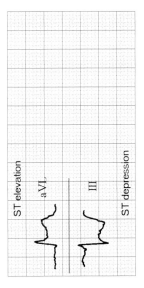

Fig. 51.2 Reciprocal changes.

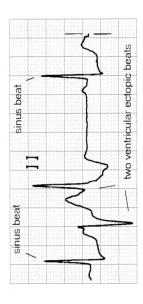

Fig. 51.3 Ectopic beats.

FEATURES OF THIS ECG

- Sinus rhythm, 66 b.p.m., normal QRS axis
- 'hyperacute' changes, indicating first few hours of infarction, in anterior leads (Fig. 51.1):
  - increased ventricular activation time (normal < 1 small square)
  - increased height of R wave
  - upsloping ST elevation
  - broad T wave with increased height
  (note V5 and V6 do not seem to fit the pattern, chest leads can be easily misplaced when in a hurry)

Causes of ST elevation

↑ Acute myocardial injury:
   – ischaemic heart disease
   – trauma
↑ Pericarditis
↑ Left bundle branch block
↑ Early repolarisation
↑ 'High take-off' especially in leads V1–3
   – apparent ST elevation after a deep S wave

CASE 52

A 67-year-old lady with 3 hours of chest pain

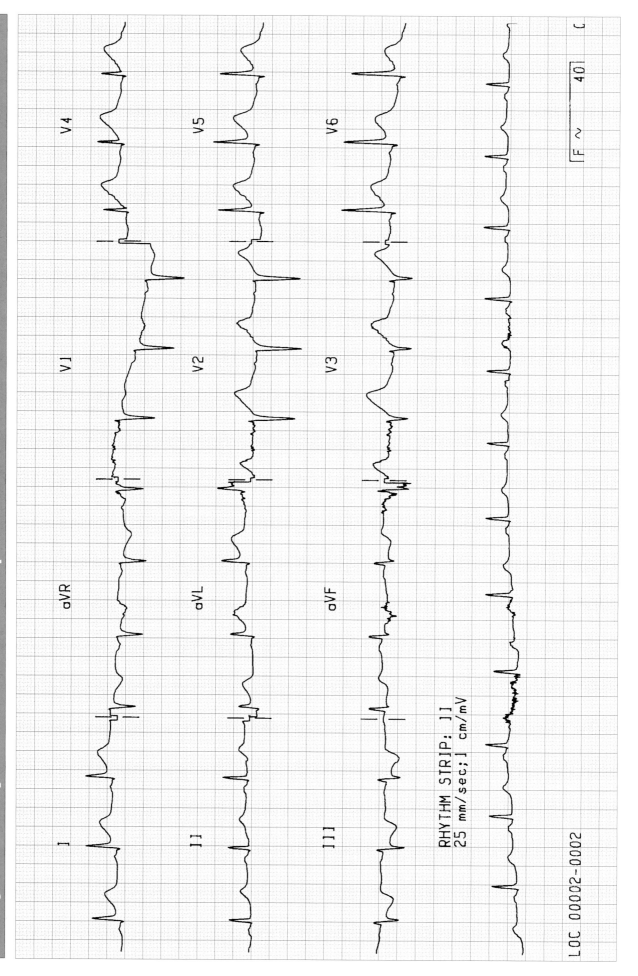

RHYTHM STRIP: II
25 mm/sec; 1 cm/mV

I

II

III

aVR

aVL

aVF

V1

V2

V3

V4

V5

V6

LOC 00002-0002

Acute anterolateral myocardial infarction

- Changes of acute injury (ST elevation) in the lateral leads V4–6, I and aVL.
- With or without reciprocal changes (ST depression) in the inferior leads.

FEATURES OF THIS ECG

- Sinus rhythm, 72 b.p.m., normal QRS axis
- Acute injury in leads V4–6, I and aVL (Fig. 52.1):
  - upsloping ST elevation
  - tall T waves
- Reciprocal ST depression in the inferior leads III and aVF (Fig. 52.2)
- Possible evidence of an old anteroseptal MI (Fig. 52.3)

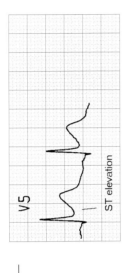

V5

ST elevation

Fig. 52.1 Acute injury.

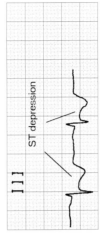

III

ST depression

Fig. 52.2 Reciprocal changes.

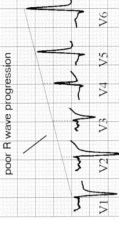

poor R wave progression

V1 V2 V3 V4 V5 V6

Fig. 52.3 Leads V1–V6.

Causes of poor R wave progression

↑ ↑ ↑ ↑ ↑ ↑ Old anteroseptal myocardial infarction
Chronic obstructive airways disease
Left ventricular hypertrophy
Left bundle branch block
Lead placement
Normal variant

CASE 53

A 50-year-old man with 7 hours of heavy chest pain

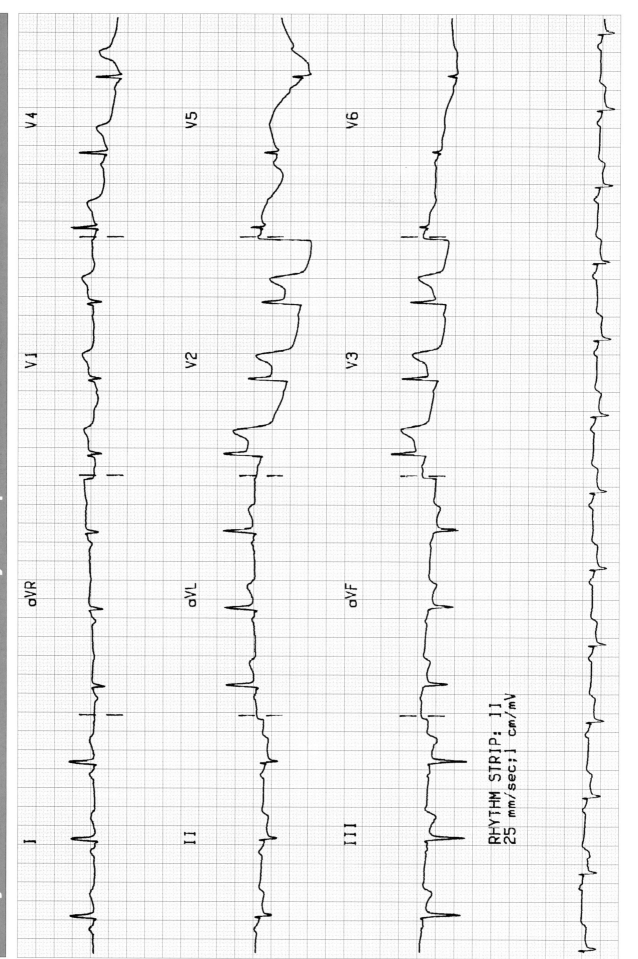

RHYTHM STRIP: II
25 mm/sec;1 cm/mV

Acute anteroseptal myocardial infarction

- Changes of acute injury (ST elevation) in the anteroseptal leads V1–4.
- With or without reciprocal changes (ST depression) in the inferolateral leads.

FEATURES OF THIS ECG

- Sinus rhythm, 78 b.p.m., left axis deviation −45°
- Acute injury in leads V1–3 (Fig. 53.I):
  - upsloping ST elevation
  - tall T waves
- Reciprocal changes in leads II, III and aVF (Fig. 53.2)

CLINICAL NOTE

At angiography this gentleman had a stenosis with thrombus in the mid-portion of his left anterior descending coronary artery. This was successfully treated with angioplasty.

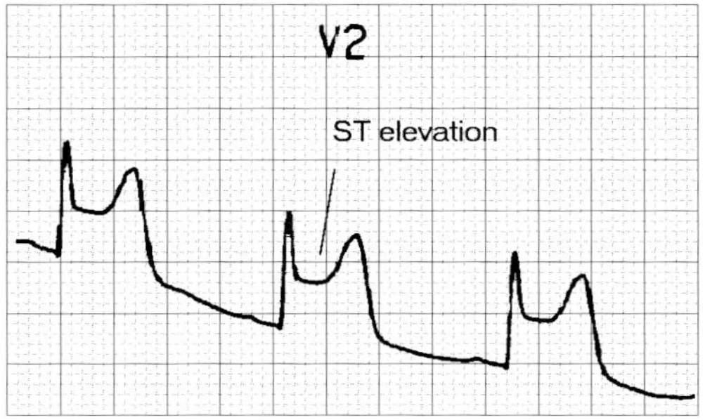

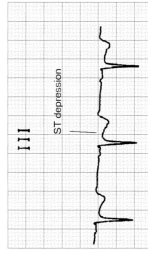

V2

ST elevation

Fig. 53.1   Acute injury.

III

ST depression

Fig. 53.2   Reciprocal changes.

CASE 54

An 83-year-old lady with acute dyspnoea

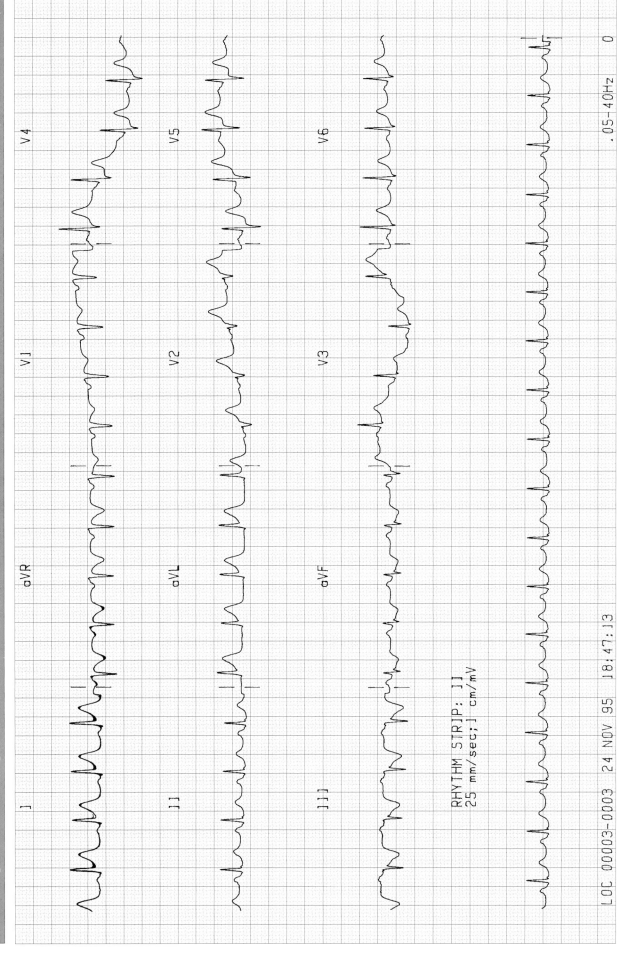

RHYTHM STRIP: II
25 mm/sec;1 cm/mV

LOC 00003-0003   24 NOV 95   18:47:13   .05-40Hz   0

Acute 'high' lateral myocardial infarction

- Changes of acute injury (ST elevation) in leads I and aVL.
- With or without reciprocal changes (ST depression) in the inferior leads.

FEATURES OF THIS ECG

- Sinus tachycardia, 108 b.p.m., normal QRS axis
- Acute injury in leads I and aVL (Fig. 54.1):
  - upsloping ST elevation
  - tall T waves
- Reciprocal ST depression in the inferior leads III and aVF (Fig. 54.2)

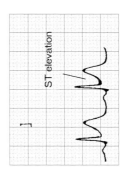

Fig. 54.1   Acute injury.

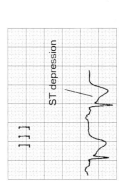

Fig. 54.2   Reciprocal changes.

CASE 55

A 56-year-old man with chest pain and vomiting for 90 minutes

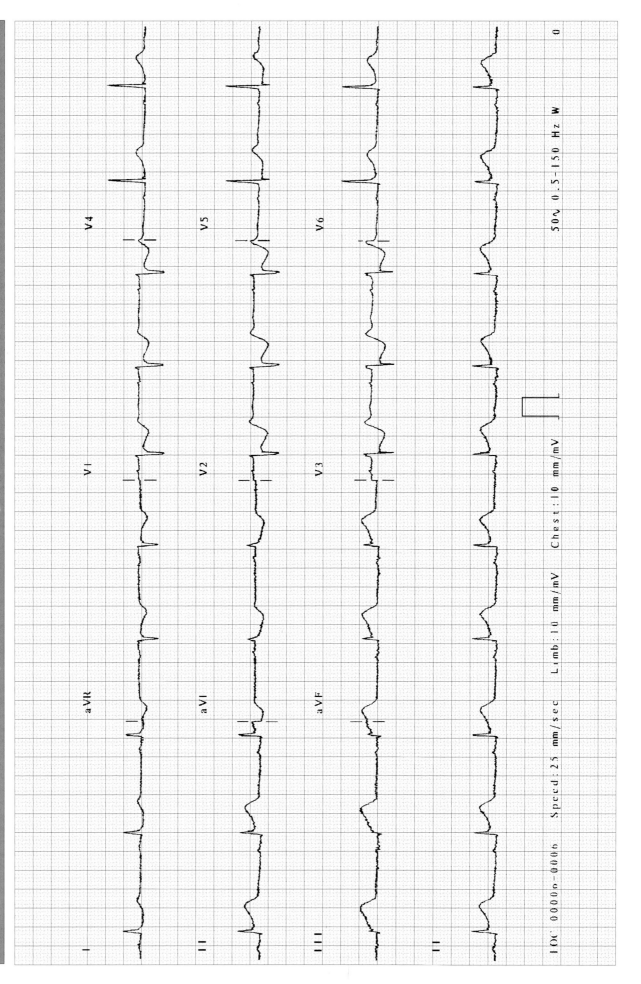

Acute inferior myocardial infarction

- Changes of acute injury (ST elevation) in the inferior leads II, III and aVF.
- With or without reciprocal changes (ST depression) in the anterior leads.

FEATURES OF THIS ECG

- Sinus rhythm, 60 b.p.m., normal QRS axis
- PR interval 200 ms, normal 120–200 ms (3–5 small squares)
- Acute injury in leads II, III and aVF (Fig. 55.1):
  - upsloping ST elevation
  - tall T waves

  These changes are also seen in lead V6 making this example an inferolateral (inferoapical) MI
- Reciprocal ST depression in the anterior leads V1–3, I and aVL (Fig. 55.2)

CLINICAL NOTE

V4R showed no ST elevation – excluding significant right ventricle infarction.

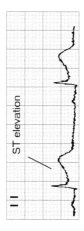

Fig. 55.1   Acute injury.

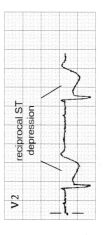

Fig. 55.2   Reciprocal changes.

CASE 56

A 54-year-old lady with 30 minutes of chest pain

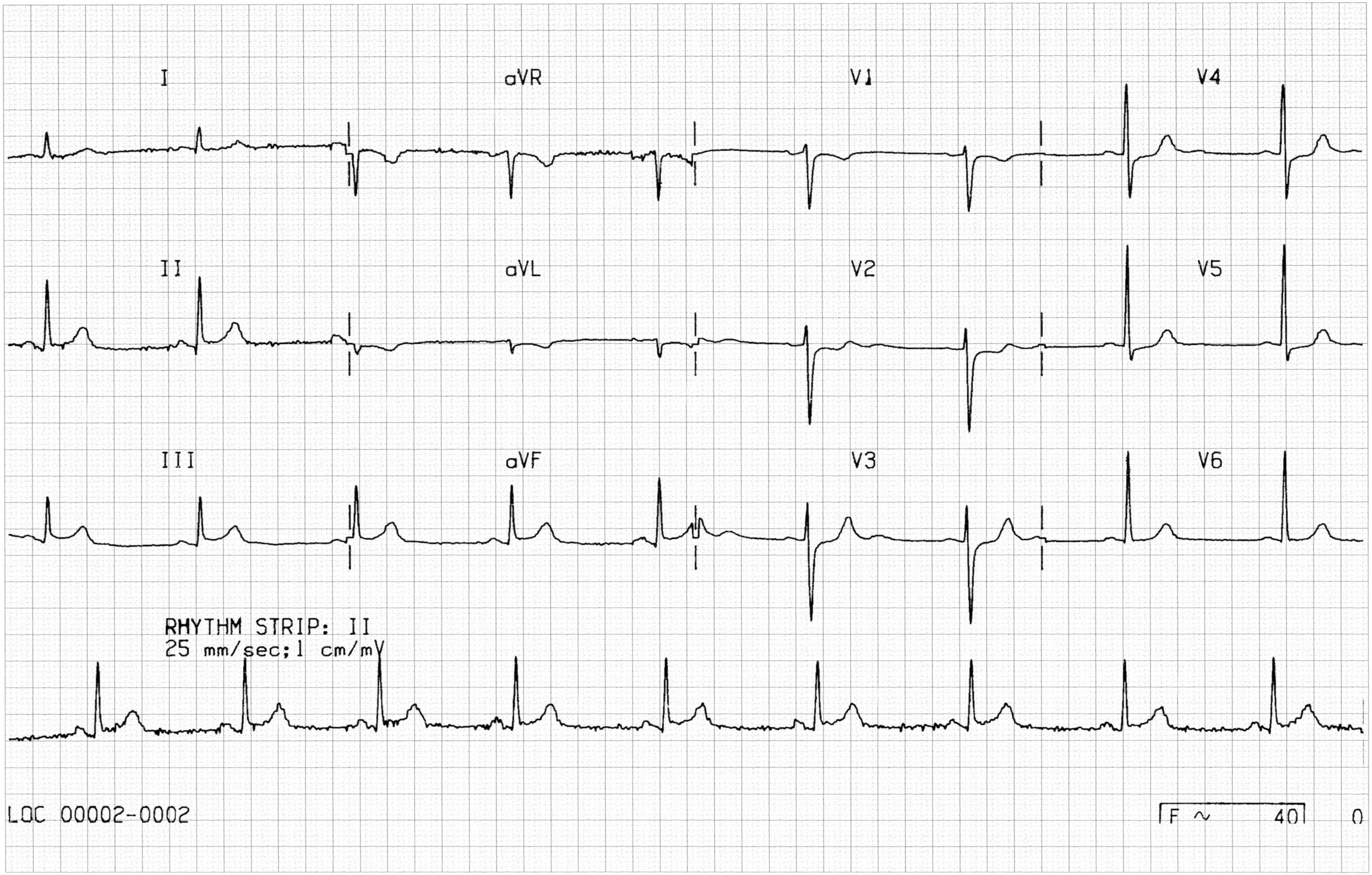

I
aVR
V1
V4

II
aVL
V2
V5

III
aVF
V3
V6

RHYTHM STRIP: II
25 mm/sec; 1 cm/mV

LOC 00002-0002

F ~ 40

Very early acute inferior myocardial infarction

The ECG features of inferior MI may appear earlier than other areas of infarction.

● Minimal changes of acute injury (ST elevation) in the inferior leads II, III and aVF with consistent reciprocal changes (ST depression) in the anterior leads.

Clinical context is important when dealing with such borderline ECGs.

FEATURES OF THIS ECG

● Sinus arrhythmia, 54 b.p.m., normal QRS axis
● Minimal ST elevation in leads II, III and aVF (Fig. 56.1)
● Suggestion of reciprocal ST depression in the anterior leads V1–4 and aVL (Fig. 56.2)

CLINICAL NOTE

This lady received thrombolysis 40 minutes after the onset of her pain.

Sometimes repeating an ECG in 30 minutes may reveal evolving diagnostic changes.

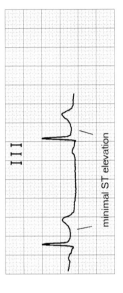

Fig. 56.1   Very early acute injury.

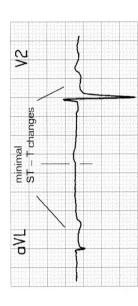

Fig. 56.2   Very early reciprocal changes.

CASE 57

A 60-year-old man with chest pain, JVP +4 cm and BP 80/50

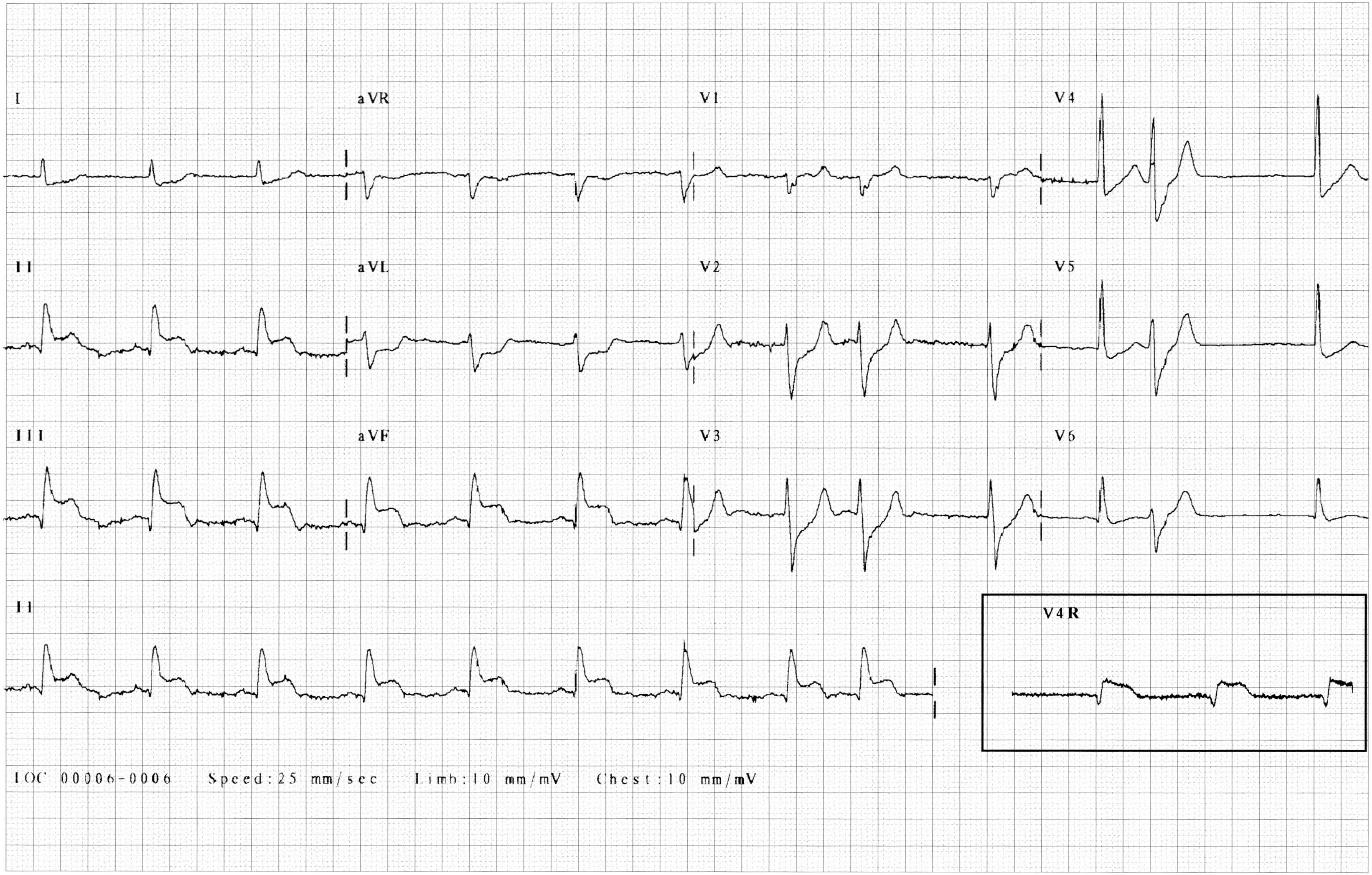

I

aVR

V1

V4

II

aVL

V2

V5

III

aVF

V3

V6

V4R

II

100 00006-0006   Speed:25 mm/sec   Limb:10 mm/mV   Chest:10 mm/mV

Acute right ventricular infarction

- ST elevation > 1 mm in lead V4R (right 5th intercostal space, mid-clavicular line).

Right ventricular infarction is most often associated with an acute inferior MI.

FEATURES OF THIS ECG

- Sinus rhythm, 78 b.p.m., normal QRS axis, incomplete RBBB
- Acute right ventricular infarction:
  – ST elevation in V4R (Fig. 57.1)
- Acute myocardial infarction (Fig. 57.2):
  – ST elevation in leads II, III and aVF
  – tall T waves
  – developing q waves
- Reciprocal ST depression in the anterior leads (Fig. 57.3)
- Junctional premature beat (JPB) (Fig. 57.4)
- Ventricular premature beat in leads V4–6

CLINICAL NOTE

Right ventricular infarction is an important reversible cause of cardiogenic shock. The first line of treatment is intravenous fluids.

Clinical features of right ventricular infarction

↑↑ Hypotension
↑↑ Clear lung fields
↑↑ Elevated JVP
↑↑ Positive Kussmaul's sign

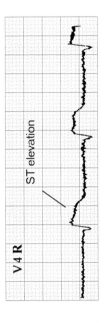

V4 R

ST elevation

Fig. 57.1   Acute injury – V4R.

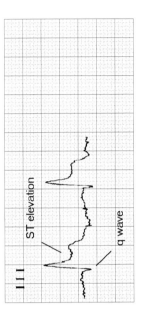

III

ST elevation

q wave

Fig. 57.2   Acute inferior MI.

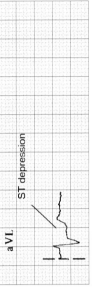

a VL.

ST depression

Fig. 57.3   Reciprocal changes.

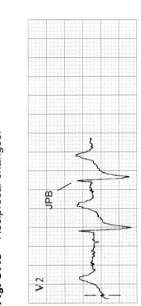

V2

JPB

Fig. 57.4   Junctional premature beat.

CASE 58

A 78-year-old lady with chest pain and collapse, BP 60/40

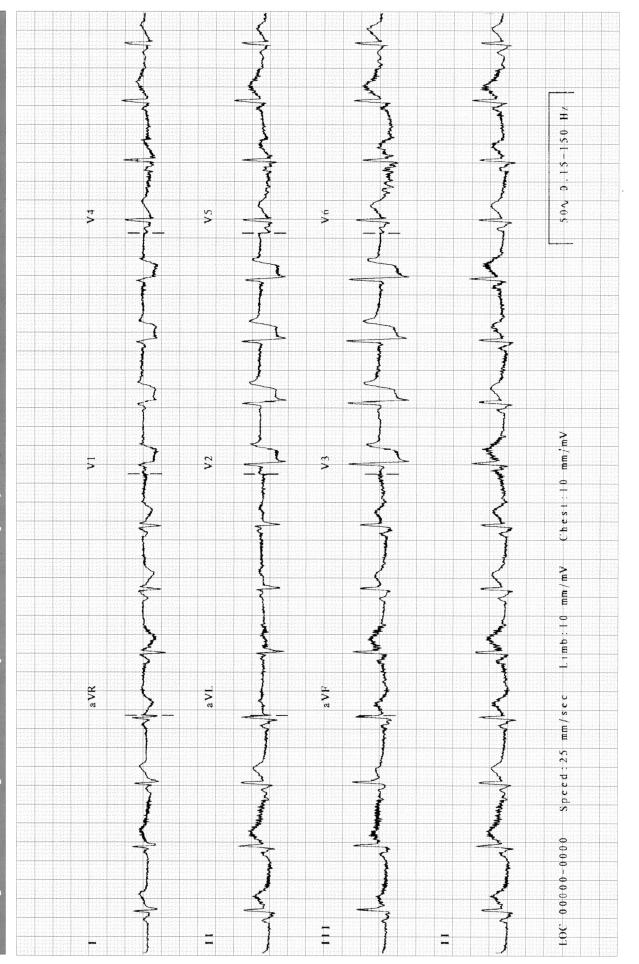

I

II

III

II

aVR

aVL

aVF

V1

V2

V3

V4

V5

V6

LOC 00-00-0000   Speed:25 mm/sec   Limb:10 mm/mV   Chest:10 mm/mV

50A 0.15-150 Hz

Acute posterior myocardial infarction

Acute posterior MI presents as the mirror image of acute injury in the septal leads since the posterior wall faces away from these leads.

- ST depression in leads V1–3.
- Prominent R wave and upright T wave in leads V1–3.

Posterior infarction is often associated with inferior and/or lateral infarction.

FEATURES OF THIS ECG

- Sinus rhythm, 90 b.p.m., normal QRS axis
- Acute posterior infarction (Fig. 58.1):
  - mirror image of acute injury in leads V1–3
- Inferolateral infarction (Fig 58.2 and 58.3):
  - ST elevation in the inferior leads (II, III and aVF)
  - ST elevation in the lateral leads V5 and 6

CLINICAL NOTE

Urgent coronary angiography, with a view to primary angioplasty, showed an occluded, dominant, left circumflex artery and infarction of the posterior, inferior and lateral regions.

This dominant left circumflex artery therefore supplied the posterior descending artery which is more commonly supplied from the right coronary artery.

Angioplasty was unsuccessful.

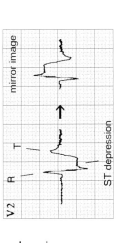

Fig. 58.1   Mirror image of acute injury.

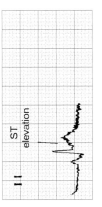

Fig. 58.2   Inferior lead.

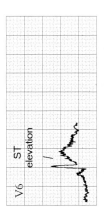

Fig. 58.3   Lateral lead.

A 74-year-old lady with severe 'crushing' chest pain for 90 minutes

Acute anterior myocardial infarction in the presence of left bundle branch block

It is often impossible to diagnose myocardial infarction with left bundle branch block (LBBB). The changes of LBBB usually mask any infarct patterns. However, about two thirds of cases may have ST–T changes.[1]

There are no reliable criteria for diagnosing infarction but there are a few pointers.

- Clinical history.
- q waves (> 30 ms) in two or more lateral leads (V5–6, I and aVL)
  - indicating anteroseptal infarction.[2]
- Primary ST and T wave changes
  - the ST and T wave changes in LBBB are called secondary changes. They are opposite to the main QRS direction. Primary changes occur in the direction of leads facing the injury. Finding ST and T wave changes in LBBB in the same direction as the QRS suggests acute injury.
- ST elevation greater than you would expect from LBBB alone
  - primary ST elevation 'adding' to the secondary ST elevation.

FEATURES OF THIS ECG

- Sinus rhythm, 80 b.p.m., left axis deviation −45°
- Left bundle branch block (Fig. 59.1):
  - broad QRS (128 ms)
  - no secondary R wave in lead V1
- Inordinate ST segment and T wave elevation in leads V2–4 (Fig. 59.2)

- Small q waves in the lateral leads I and aVL (Fig. 59.3)
  – not diagnostic

CLINICAL NOTE

Serial cardiac enzymes confirmed the diagnosis of acute myocardial infarction.

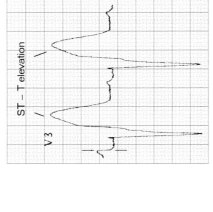

Fig. 59.2 Inordinate ST–T changes.

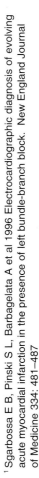

Fig. 59.1 Left bundle branch block.

Fig. 59.3 Small lateral q waves.

[1] Sgarbossa E B, Pinski S L, Barbagelata A et al 1996 Electrocardiographic diagnosis of evolving acute myocardial infarction in the presence of left bundle-branch block. New England Journal of Medicine 334: 481–487

[2] Rhoades D V et al 1961 The electrocardiogram in the presence of myocardial infarction and intraventricular block of the left bundle-branch type. American Heart Journal 62: 735

HYPERTROPHY PATTERNS

- Right atrial abnormality (P-pulmonale)
- Left atrial abnormality (P-mitrale)
- Biatrial hypertrophy
- Right ventricular hypertrophy (RVH)
- Left ventricular hypertrophy (LVH)

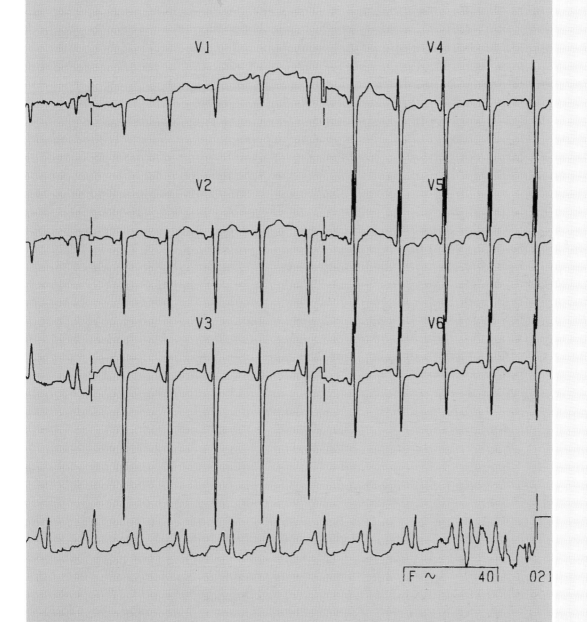

CASE 60

A 54-year-old lady with bronchiectasis

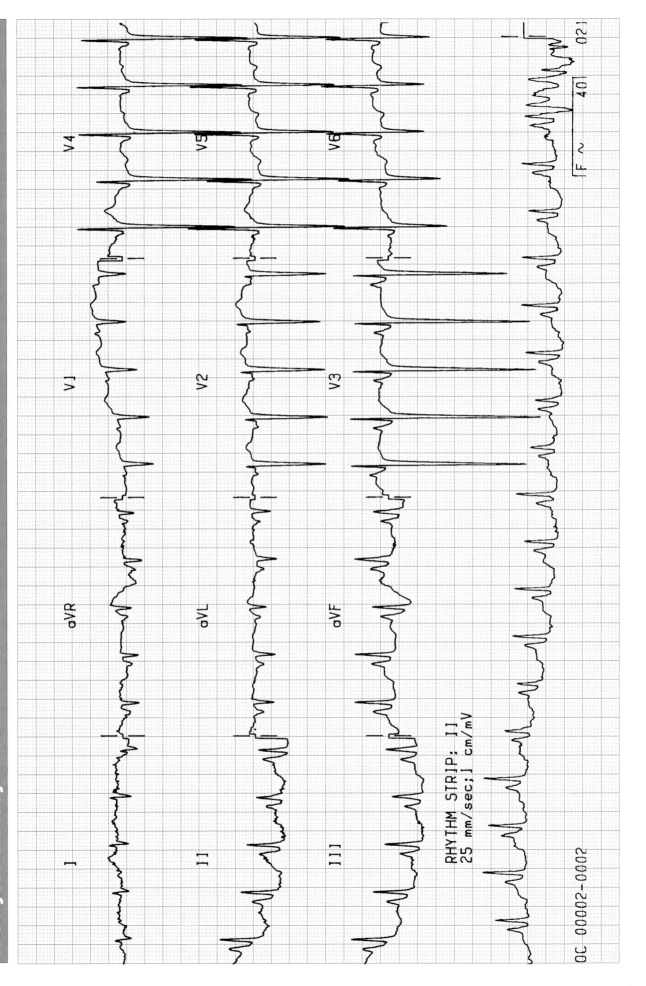

I

aVR

V1

V4

II

aVL

V2

V5

III

aVF

V3

V6

RHYTHM STRIP: II
25 mm/sec; 1 cm/mV

0C 00002-0002

Right atrial abnormality (P-pulmonale)

- P waves more than 3 mm in height in leads II, III, or aVF.

- Other features:
  - tall P waves in the right chest leads (> 1.5 mm)
  - prominent atrial repolarisation (Ta) wave.

FEATURES OF THIS ECG

- Sinus tachycardia, 120 b.p.m., rightward QRS axis
- Diagnostic features of P-pulmonale:
  - abnormally tall P waves in II, III, and aVF (Fig. 60.1)
  - tall P wave in lead V3 (Fig. 60.2)
  - prominent Ta wave (Fig. 60.2)
- Features of chronic obstructive airways disease:
  - clockwise electrical rotation (late transition)
  - posterior displacement of the QRS axis (deep S waves in the right chest leads)

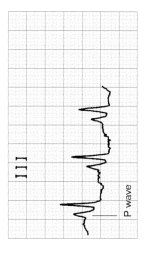

Fig. 60.1 P-pulmonale.

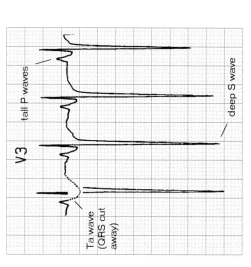

Fig. 60.2 Ta wave.

Causes of right atrial abnormality

↑ Raised right ventricular pressure:
  - pulmonary hypertension from any cause
  - cor pulmonale
↑ Tricuspid valve stenosis
↑ Right atrial ischaemia or infarction (uncommon)

CASE 61

A 43-year-old Maori man with a diastolic murmur

Left atrial abnormality (P-mitrale)

- Notched P wave which exceeds 120 ms (3 small squares) in duration in leads I, II, aVF or aVL.

- Other features:
  - terminal negative component to the P wave in V1.

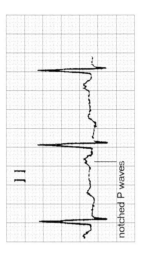

notched P waves

Fig. 61.1 P-mitrale.

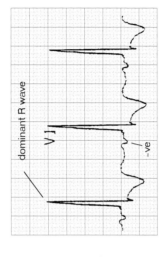

dominant R wave

V1

-ve

Fig. 61.2 Lead V1.

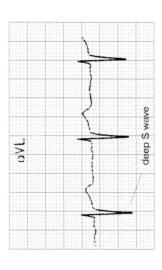

aVL

deep S wave

Fig. 61.3 Lead aVL.

FEATURES OF THIS ECG

- Sinus rhythm, 72 b.p.m., vertical QRS axis
- Features of P-mitrale:
  - broad, notched P waves seen in the inferior leads (Fig. 61.1)
  - negative component to P wave in lead V1 (Fig. 61.2)
- Features of right ventricular hypertrophy:
  - dominant R wave in lead V1, with ST depression and T wave inversion (Fig. 61.2)
  - deep S waves in the lateral leads (Fig. 61.3)

CLINICAL NOTE

The combination of left atrial hypertrophy and right ventricular hypertrophy suggests mitral stenosis. This patient had mitral stenosis on the basis of rheumatic heart disease.

Causes of left atrial abnormality

→ Systemic hypertension
→ Left ventricular failure
→ Aortic or mitral valve disease

CASE 62

A 24-year-old lady with a history of rheumatic fever

Biatrial hypertrophy

- P waves in the limb leads more than 3 mm in height and also greater than 120 ms (3 small squares) in duration.
- Large biphasic P waves in V1 with an initial positive deflection of more than 2 mm and a terminal negative portion at least 1 mm deep and 40 ms (1 small square) in duration.
- P wave greater than 2 mm in height in V1 in combination with notched P waves, greater than 120 ms in duration in the limb leads or left precordial leads.

Any of these three criteria suggests the diagnosis of biatrial hypertrophy.

FEATURES OF THIS ECG

- Sinus rhythm, 92 b.p.m., vertical QRS axis
- Features of biatrial hypertrophy:
  - P waves in the limb leads which are broad, notched, and tall (Fig. 62.1)
  - large biphasic P wave in V1 (Fig. 62.2)
  - notched P waves with a duration of greater than 120 ms in the left precordial leads (Fig. 62.3)
- Long PR interval, greater than 200 ms (Fig. 62.4)

CLINICAL NOTE

This lady had rheumatic triple valve disease. Her cardiac catheter study documented critical tricuspid stenosis, severe mitral stenosis, and severe aortic stenosis.

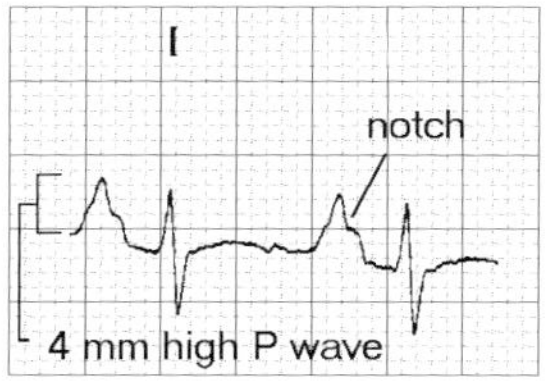

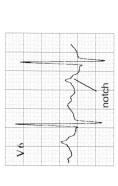

Fig. 62.1 Lead I.

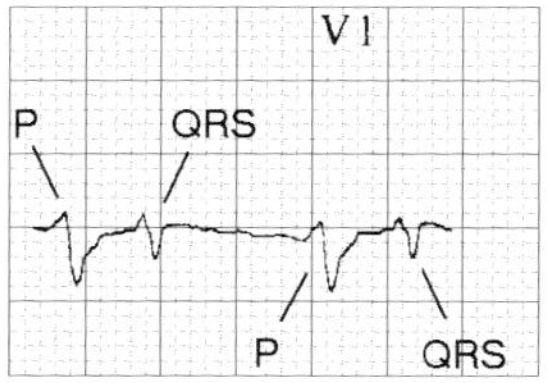

Fig. 62.2 Large biphasic P waves.

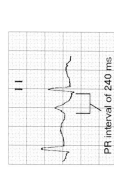

Fig. 62.3 Lead V6.

Fig. 62.4 Long PR interval.

A 25-year-old lady with Down syndrome

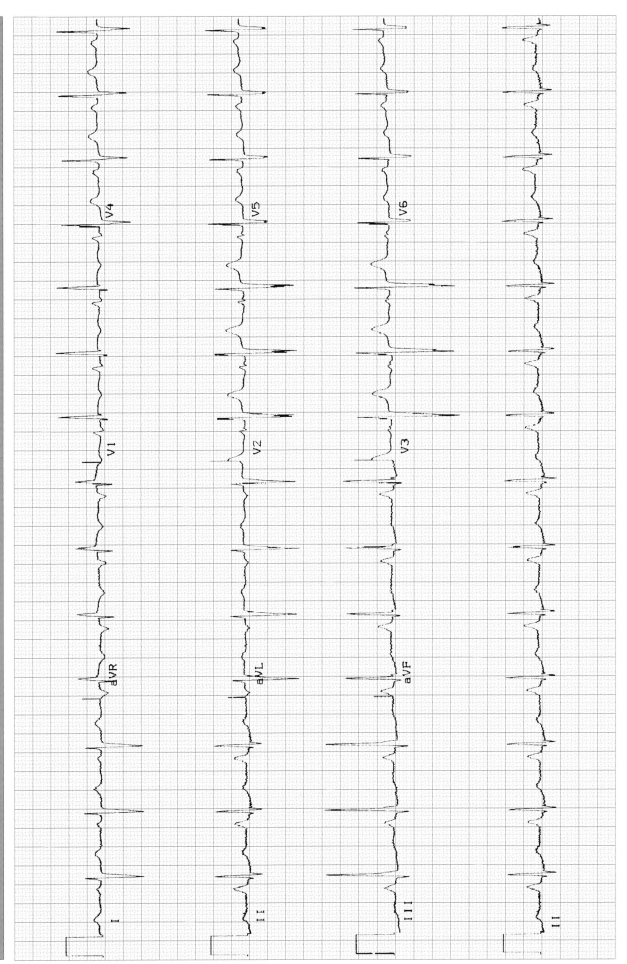

Right ventricular hypertrophy (RVH)

- Right axis deviation (QRS axis > +90°).
- Dominant R wave in V1.
- No evidence of anterolateral myocardial infarction or bundle branch block.
- Other features:
  - ST segment depression and T wave inversion in the right chest leads (V1–4)
  - deep S waves in the lateral leads (V4–6, I and aVL).

right-to-left shunt (Eisenmenger syndrome). She was deeply cyanosed and died several days after this ECG was taken.

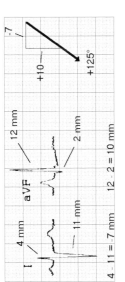

4 - 11 = -7 mm   12 - 2 = 10 mm

Fig. 63.1 Right axis deviation.

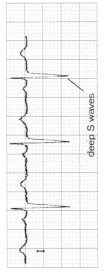

Fig. 63.2 Lead V1.

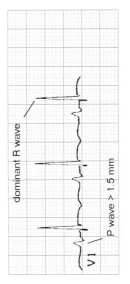

Fig. 63.3 Lead I.

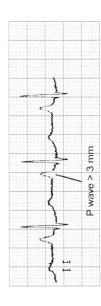

Fig. 63.4 P-pulmonale.

FEATURES OF THIS ECG

- Sinus rhythm, 84 b.p.m.
- Features of RVH:
  - right axis deviation, +125° (Fig. 63.1)
  - dominant R wave in V1 (Fig. 63.2)
  - deep S waves in the lateral leads (Fig. 63.3)
- Features of right atrial hypertrophy:
  - abnormally tall P waves in the inferior leads and V1 (Figs 63.2 and 63.4)

CLINICAL NOTE

This lady had a congenital ventricular septal defect with a large

Causes of a dominant R wave in V1

↑ Normal finding in children
↑ Right ventricular hypertrophy
↑ Right bundle branch block
↑ True posterior myocardial infarction
↑ Ventricular pre-excitation
↑ Duchenne muscular dystrophy

CASE 64

A 25-year-old male soccer player with an ejection systolic murmur

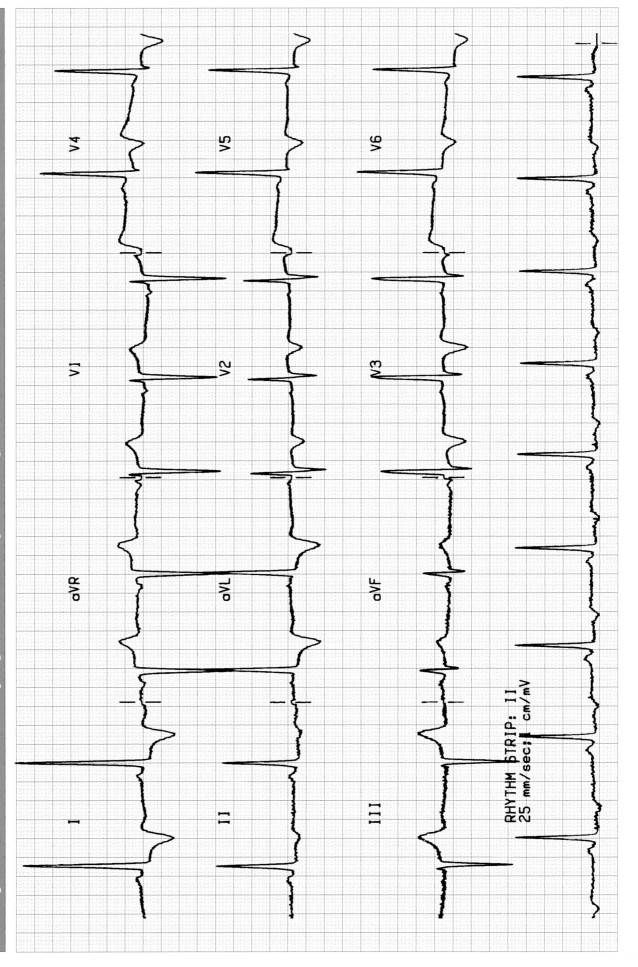

I   aVR   V1   V4

II   aVL   V2   V5

III   aVF   V3   V6

RHYTHM STRIP: II
25 mm/sec; 1 cm/mV

Left ventricular hypertrophy (LVH)

- There are a number of criteria for LVH based on the voltages of the QRS deflections (see criteria listed below). These criteria have good specificity but poor sensitivity.

- Other features:
  - ST depression and T wave inversion (LV strain pattern) in leads with prominent R waves
  - counterclockwise electrical rotation (early transition)
  - increased ventricular activation time
  - inverted U waves in the left chest leads
  - leftward QRS axis.

Voltage criteria for LVH

Sokolow & Lyon:[1]	SV1 + R(V5 or V6) > 35 mm
Cornell:[2]	SV3 + RaVL > 28 mm in men
	SV3 + RaVL > 20 mm in women
Framingham:[3]	RaVL > 11 mm
	RV4–6 > 25 mm
	SV1–3 > 25 mm
	S(V1 or V2) + R(V5 or V6) > 35 mm
	RI + SIII > 25 mm
Romhilt & Estes:[4]	Point score system

FEATURES OF THIS ECG

- Sinus bradycardia, 54 b.p.m.
- Features of LVH (Fig. 64.1):
  - leftward axis
  - early electrical transition (dominant R in V2)
  - tall R waves in aVL and lead I
  - tall R waves in the left chest leads and deep S wave in V1
  - widespread ST depression and T wave inversion

CLINICAL NOTE

Hypertrophic obstructive cardiomyopathy (HOCM) was diagnosed at echocardiography.

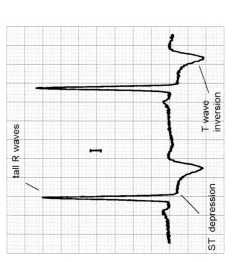

Fig. 64.1   Lead I.

[1] Sokolow M, Lyon T P 1949 Ventricular complex in left ventricular hypertrophy as obtained by unipolar precordial and limb leads. American Heart Journal 37: 161
[2] Casale P N et al 1987 Improved sex-specific criteria for left ventricular hypertrophy for clinical and computer interpretation of electrocardiograms: validation with autopsy findings. Circulation 75 (3): 565–572
[3] Levy D et al 1990 Determinants of sensitivity and specificity of electrocardiographic criteria for left ventricular hypertrophy. Circulation 81: 815–820
[4] Romhilt D W, Estes E H 1986 Point score system for the ECG diagnosis of left ventricular hypertrophy. American Heart Journal 75: 752–758

MISCELLANEOUS

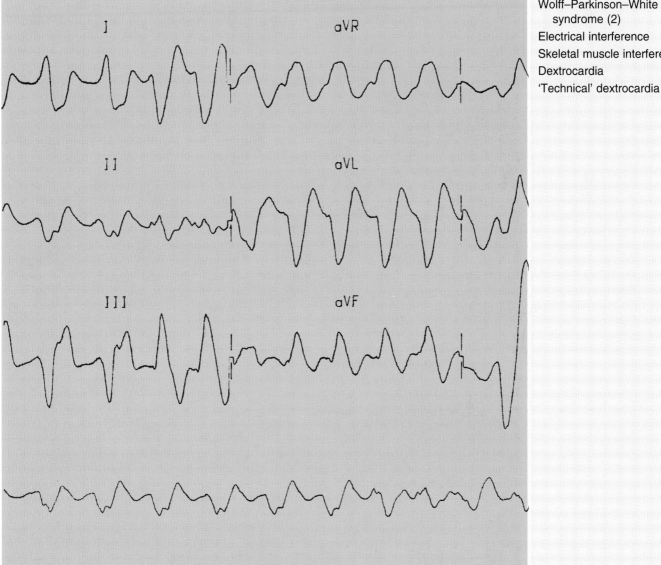

CASE 65

A 21-year-old male pilot

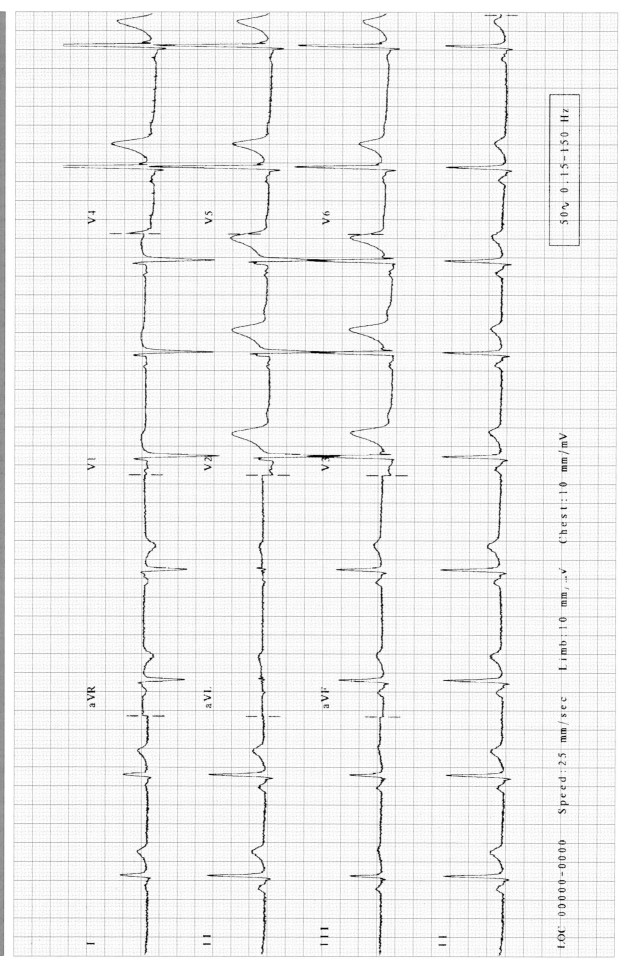

aVR

aVL

aVF

V1

V2

V3

V4

V5

V6

I

II

III

II

LOC:00000-0000   Speed:25 mm/sec   Limb:10 mm/mV   Chest:10 mm/mV

50~ 0.15-150 Hz

The athletic heart

Young athletic hearts may show the following features:

- 'early repolarisation':
  - prominent J waves best seen in leads V5–6
  - concave upward, minimally elevated ST segments
- relatively tall, frequently symmetrical T waves
  - (T waves are usually asymmetrical)
- occasionally inverted T waves laterally
- prominent mid-precordial U waves
- prominent, but narrow, q waves in the left precordial leads
- sinus bradycardia
- persistent juvenile pattern – T wave inversion V1–3
- left ventricular hypertrophy voltage criteria.

FEATURES OF THIS ECG

- Sinus arrhythmia, rate 54 b.p.m., normal QRS axis
- Features of an athletic heart (Fig 65.1):
  - narrow q waves
  - early repolarisation V2–6
  - symmetrical T waves
  - U waves
  - large voltage deflections

CLINICAL NOTE

This young man was a cross country runner and physical education instructor.

An echocardiogram showed concentric left ventricular hypertrophy.

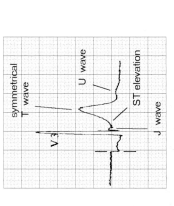

Fig. 65.1 Athletic heart.

CASE 66

A thin 79-year-old lady found on the floor at home

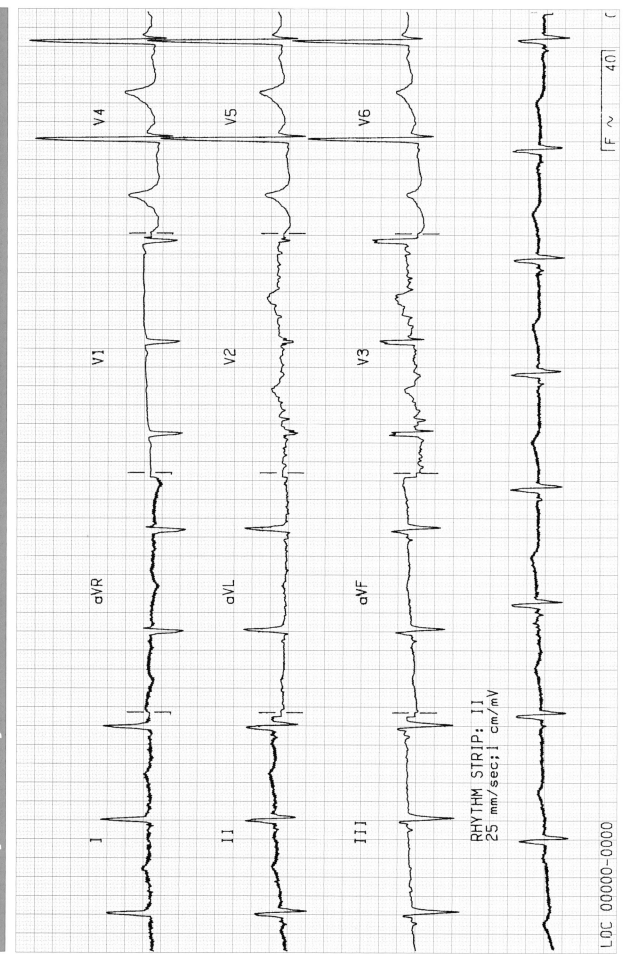

RHYTHM STRIP: II
25 mm/sec;1 cm/mV

LOC 00000-0000

SECTION 8

147

CASE 66

Hypothermia

- Bradycardia.
- Prominent deflection at the junction of QRS and ST segment (J wave)
  - an extreme example, from another patient, is shown in Figure 66.1, temperature = 26°C.
- Increased ventricular activation time.
- Long QT interval.
- Shivering artifact.

Fig. 66.1 Hypothermia.

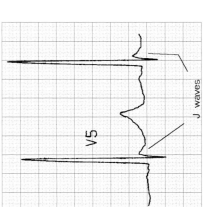

Fig. 66.2 J waves.

FEATURES OF THIS ECG

- Bradycardia, 48 b.p.m.
- Prominent J waves in leads V4–6 (Fig. 66.2)
- A shivering artifact is seen in leads V2 and V3.
- Left anterior hemiblock:
  - left axis deviation –36°
  - initial R waves in the inferior leads

CLINICAL NOTE

This lady had a core temperature of 27°C.

CASE 67

A 52-year-old man with marked weakness of both arms and legs

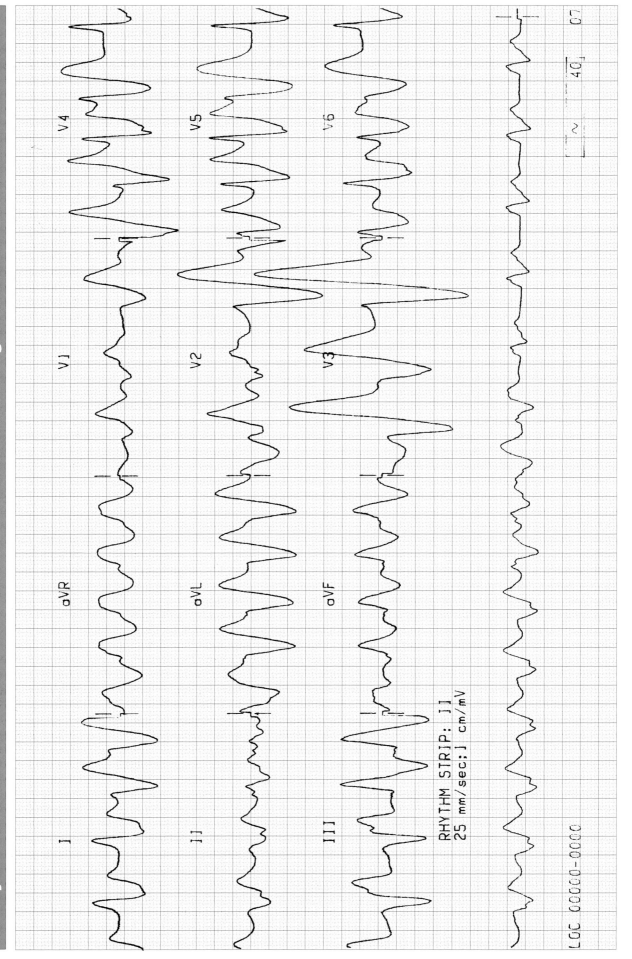

RHYTHM STRIP: II
25 mm/sec; 1 cm/mV

LOC 00000-0000

Hyperkalaemia

- Small or absent p waves.
- Long PR interval.
- Atrial fibrillation.
- Broad QRS complexes especially the terminal component.
- Decreased R wave size.
- Axis deviation.
- Shortened or absent ST segment.
- Tall tented T waves ('they would hurt if you sat on them!').
- Ventricular fibrillation.

FEATURES OF THIS ECG

- Indeterminate rhythm, 90 b.p.m., right axis deviation
- Broad, bizarre complexes (Fig. 67.1)
- Towards the end of the rhythm strip there are features suggestive of hyperkalaemia (Fig. 67.2)

CLINICAL NOTE

This man was on haemodialysis and had gone on a long fishing trip. Hyperkalaemia causes muscular weakness as well as cardiac arrhythmias.

The serum potassium was 10.1 mmol/l and an injection of calcium gluconate led to a return of a P wave, narrowing of the QRS complex, return of an ST segment and a T wave that looked more typical of hyperkalaemia (Fig. 67.3).

Common causes of severe hyperkalaemia

↑ Acute or chronic renal failure
↑ Tissue damage, e.g. crush injury or post-cardiac arrest
↑ Drugs: potassium-sparing diuretics, ACE inhibitors

After haemodialysis an obvious P wave and narrow QRS had returned. (Fig. 67.4).

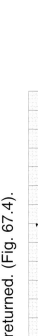
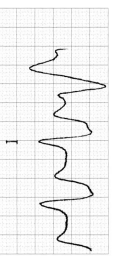

Fig. 67.1   K⁺ = 10.1 mmol/l.

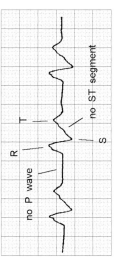

Fig. 67.2   Rhythm strip.

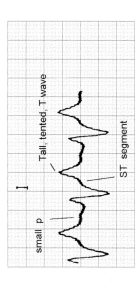

Fig. 67.3   10 minutes after Ca⁺⁺.

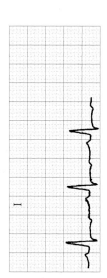

Fig. 67.4   After haemodialysis K⁺ = 5.3 mmol/l.

CASE 68

A 19-year-old girl with weakness and falls

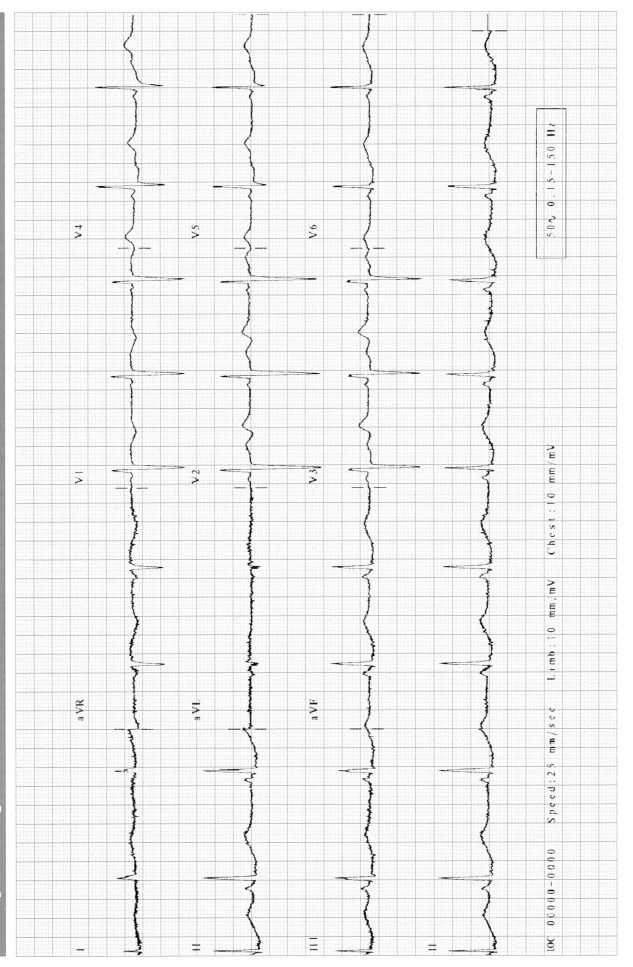

LOC 00000-0000   Speed:25 mm/sec   Limb:10 mm/mV   Chest:10 mm/mV

50∿ 0.15–150 Hz

Hypokalaemia

- Small or absent T waves.
- Prominent U waves.
- Long PR interval.
- ST segment depression.

FEATURES OF THIS ECG

- Sinus rhythm, 60 b.p.m., normal QRS axis
- Changes of hypokalaemia (Fig. 68.1):
  – prominent U waves
  – small T waves
  – minimal ST depression (Fig. 68.2)

Hypokalaemia may give the false impression of a long QT interval (Fig. 68.2). It is actually a QU interval!

CLINICAL NOTE

This young lady had bulimia and had been making herself vomit. Her serum potassium was 1.6 mmol/l.

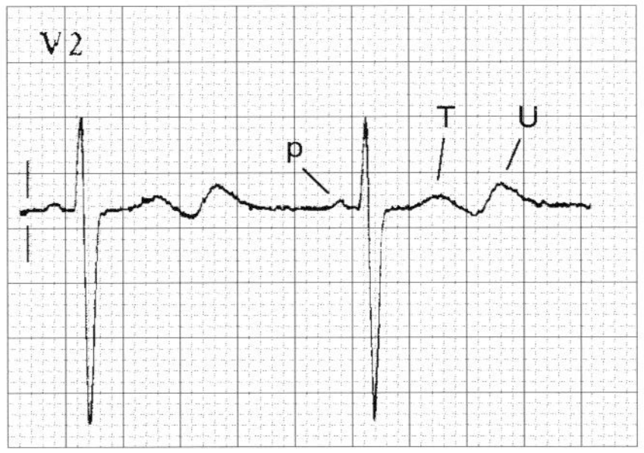

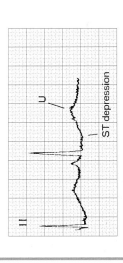

Fig. 68.1 Lead V2.

Fig. 68.2 Lead II.

Common causes of hypokalaemia

→ Gastrointestinal losses:
  – vomiting
  – diarrhoea
→ Drugs:
  – diuretics
  – corticosteroids
  – bronchodilators
  – laxatives

A 55-year-old lady with back pain

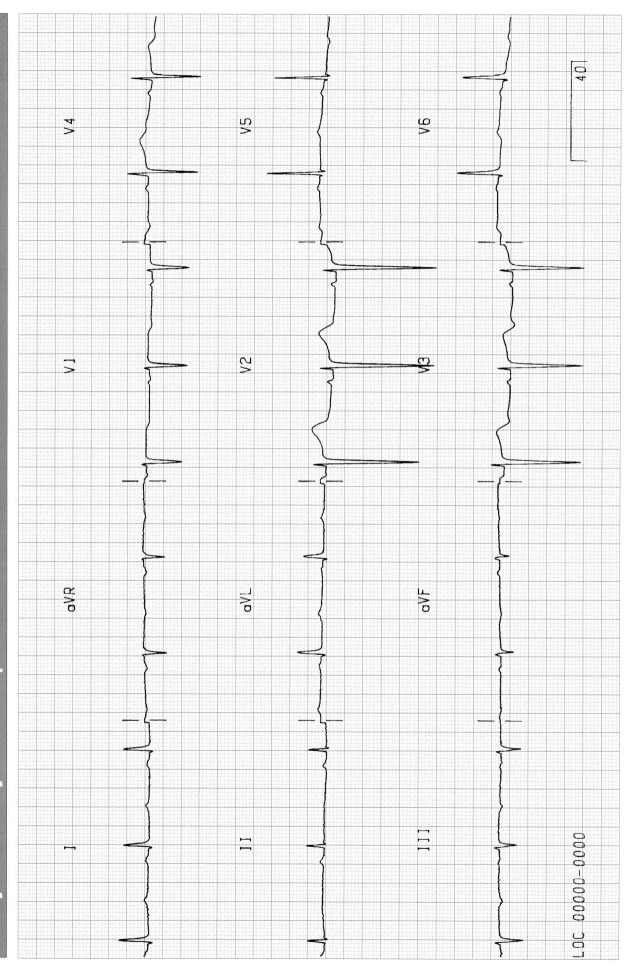

I

aVR

V1

V4

II

aVL

V2

V5

III

aVF

V3

V6

40

LOC 00000-0000

Hypocalcaemia

- Long QT interval due to prolonged ST segment.
- ST segment tends to 'hug' the baseline.
- T wave may be small and symmetrical.

FEATURES OF THIS ECG

- Sinus rhythm, 60 b.p.m., normal QRS axis
- Features of hypocalcaemia (Fig. 69.1):
  – long ST segment and QT interval
  – no displacement of the ST segment

CLINICAL NOTE

This lady had a serum calcium of 1.7 mmol/l and was shown to have vitamin D deficiency.

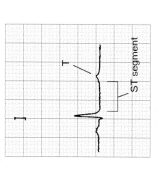

Fig. 69.1 Lead I.

Common causes of hypocalcaemia

↑↑ Elderly and housebound
↑↑ Chronic diarrhoea
↑↑ Anticonvulsant drugs
↑↑ Chronic renal failure
↑↑ Hypoparathyroidism

CASE 70

A 46-year-old lady with polyuria and polydipsia

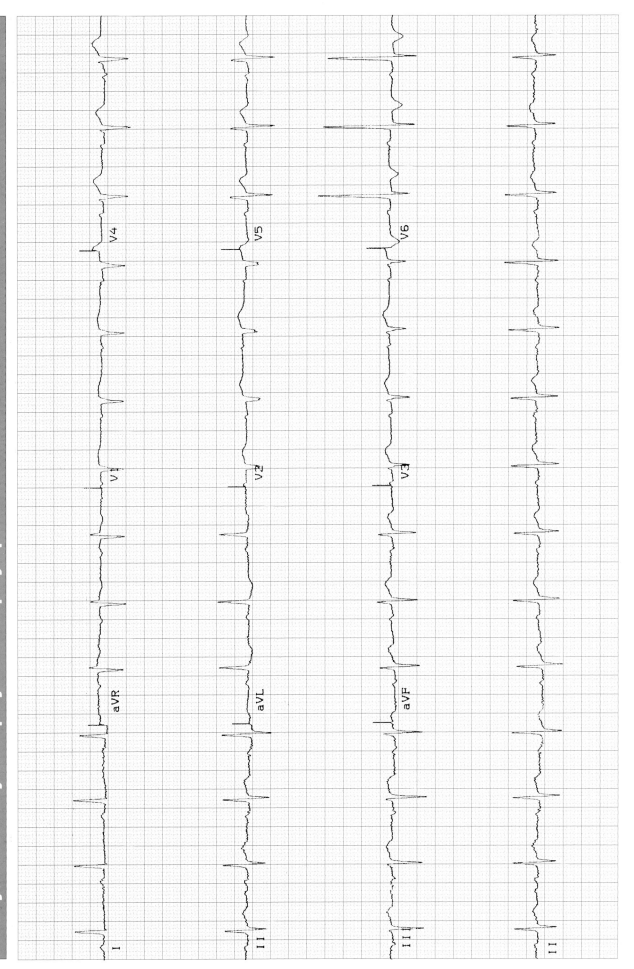

Hypercalcaemia

- A short QT interval due to a short or absent ST segment.
- The distal limb of the T wave may be steeper than the proximal.

FEATURES OF THIS ECG

- Sinus rhythm, 84 b.p.m., leftward QRS axis –20°
- Features of hypercalcaemia (Fig. 70.1):
  - very short ST segment
  - corrected QT interval of 390 ms (normal 440 ms)
- Non-specific lateral T wave changes (Fig. 70.2)

CLINICAL NOTE

The serum calcium was 3.5 mmol/l and this lady was shown to have primary hyperparathyroidism. She also suffered from hypertension.

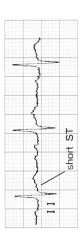

Fig. 70.1 Lead II.

short ST

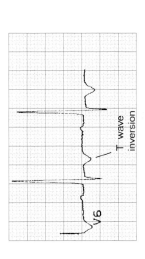

Fig. 70.2 Lead V6.

T wave inversion

V6

Causes of a short corrected QT interval

↑ Hypercalcaemia
↑ Hyperthermia
↑ Digoxin effect
↑ Vagal stimulation

CASE 71

A 60-year-old man with dyspnoea and BP 90/60

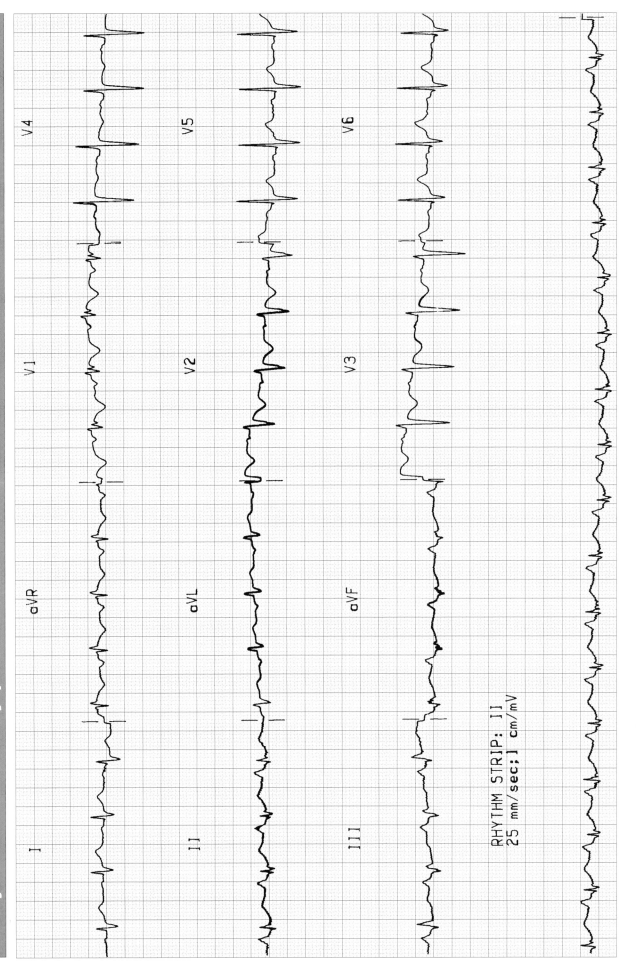

I

aVR

V1

V4

II

aVL

V2

V5

III

aVF

V3

V6

RHYTHM STRIP: II
25 mm/sec; 1 cm/mV

Acute pulmonary embolus

In massive pulmonary embolus the following, often transient, changes may be seen:

- an S1 Q3 T3 pattern
- sinus tachycardia
- incomplete or complete RBBB
- T wave inversion in leads V1–V3.

Other changes seen:
- Prominent R wave in lead aVR
- Prominent S wave in lead V6
- Low amplitude deflections.

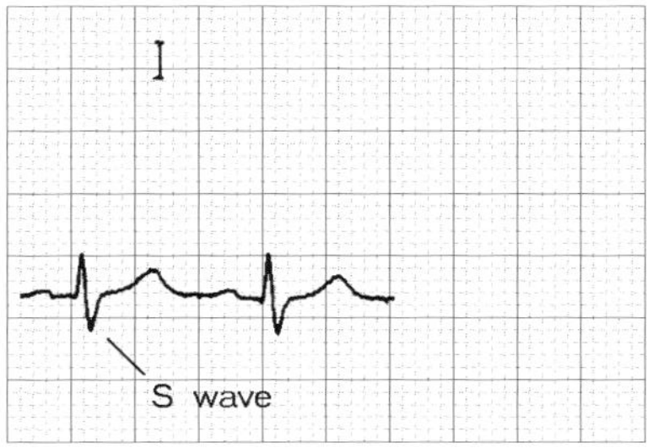

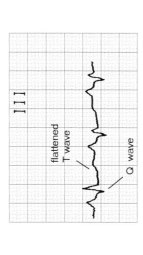

Fig. 71.1 S1.

Fig. 71.2 Q3 T3.

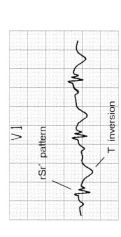

Fig. 71.3 Lead V1.

FEATURES OF THIS ECG

- Sinus tachycardia, 102 b.p.m., superior axis −90° (or +270°)
- Features of acute pulmonary embolus:
  - prominent S wave in lead I (Fig. 71.1)
  - Q wave and T wave changes in lead III (Fig. 71.2)
  - incomplete RBBB pattern (Fig. 71.3)
  - T wave inversion in the right-sided chest leads (Fig. 71.3)
  - sinus tachycardia

CLINICAL NOTE

This man had a massive pulmonary embolus but recovered well.

Causes of an S1 Q3 T3 pattern

→ Normal variant
→ Acute pulmonary embolus
→ Left posterior hemiblock

A 53-year-old man with pleuritic chest pain 1 week after an MI

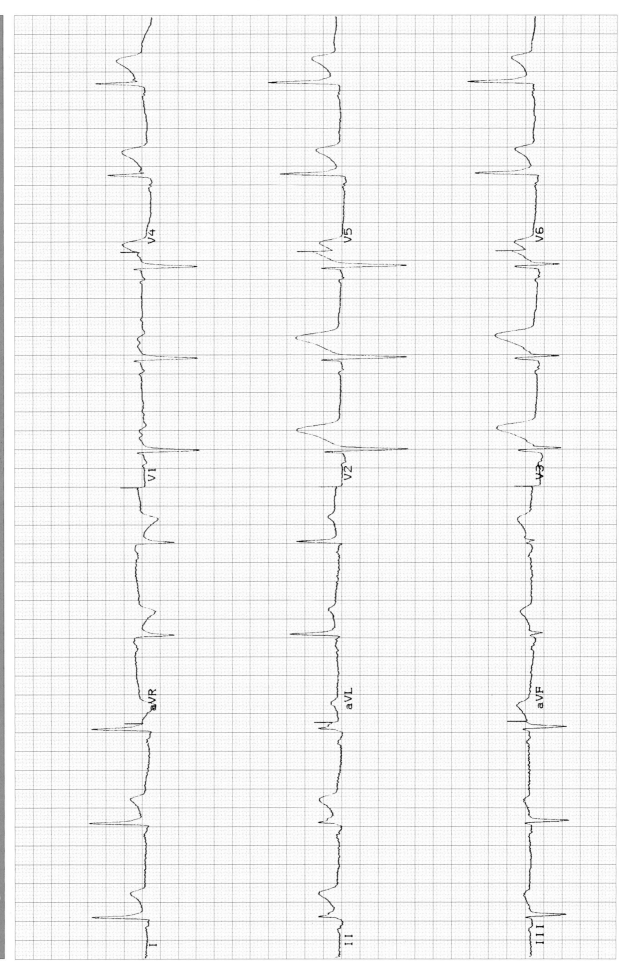

Pericarditis

- Concave upwards, 'saddle-shaped', ST elevation in multiple leads.
- Tall T waves.

Classically, leads V4–6 and II show the most prominent ST elevation and aVR shows ST depression.

FEATURES OF THIS ECG

- Sinus rhythm, rate 60 b.p.m., normal QRS axis
- ST elevation in the inferior leads (Fig. 72.1) and anterior leads with a concave upwards appearance

CLINICAL NOTE

This man had Dressler's syndrome which resolved over a few days.

Fig. 72.1 Lead II.

Common causes of pericarditis

- → Viral
- → Myocardial infarction
- → Malignancy
- → Uraemia
- → TB
- → Dressler's syndrome
- → Connective tissue disease
- → Hypothyroidism

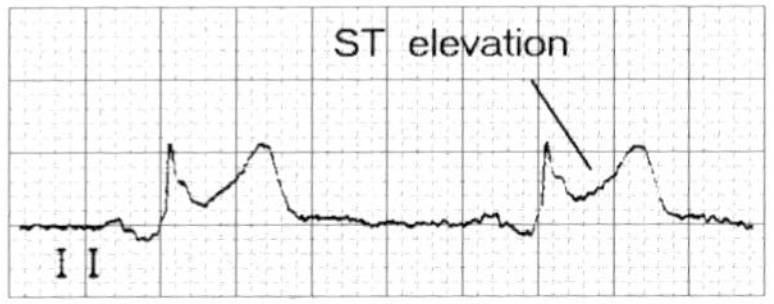

A 38-year-old breathless lady with raised JVP and Kussmaul's sign

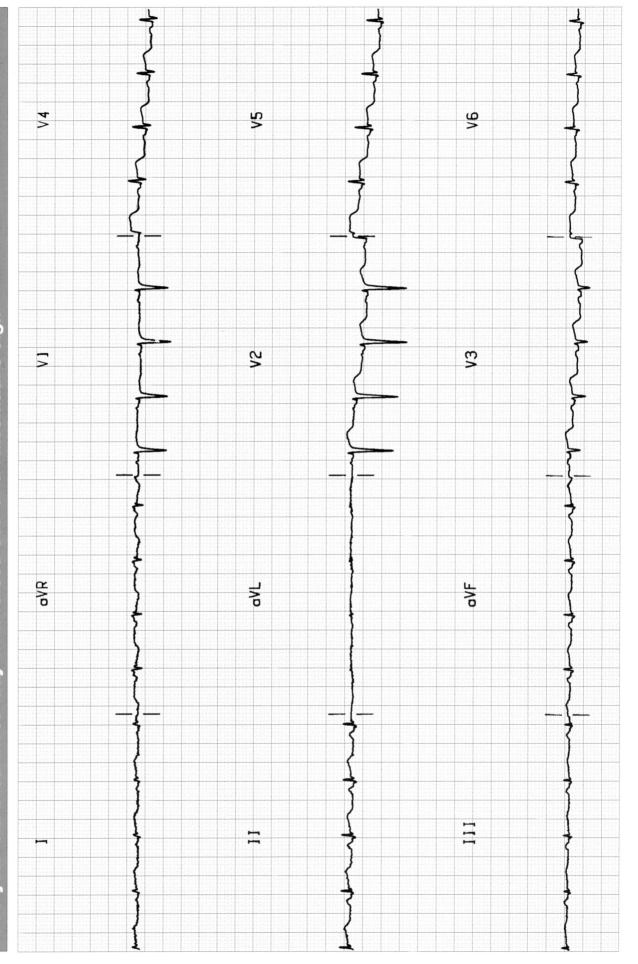

Pericardial effusion

- Small voltage deflections.
- Low or inverted T waves.

FEATURES OF THIS ECG

- Sinus tachycardia, 108 b.p.m., normal QRS axis
- Small deflections suggesting pericardial effusion (Fig. 73.1)
- Minimal ST elevation in the anterior (Fig. 73.2) and inferior leads suggesting pericarditis

CLINICAL NOTE

This lady had pericardial tamponade due to pericarditis related to systemic sclerosis. 200 ml of straw coloured fluid was drained with immediate clinical improvement.

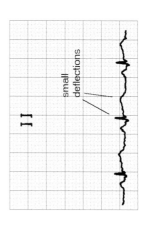

Fig. 73.1 Lead II.

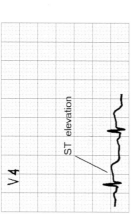

Fig. 73.2 Lead V4.

Causes of small QRS complexes

↑ Obesity
↑ Large breasts
↑ Silicone breast implant
↑ Pericardial effusion (shown here)
↑ Left pleural effusion
↑ Chronic obstructive airways disease
↑ Acute pulmonary embolus
↑ Hypothyroidism

CASE 74

A 14-year-old unconscious girl with dilated pupils

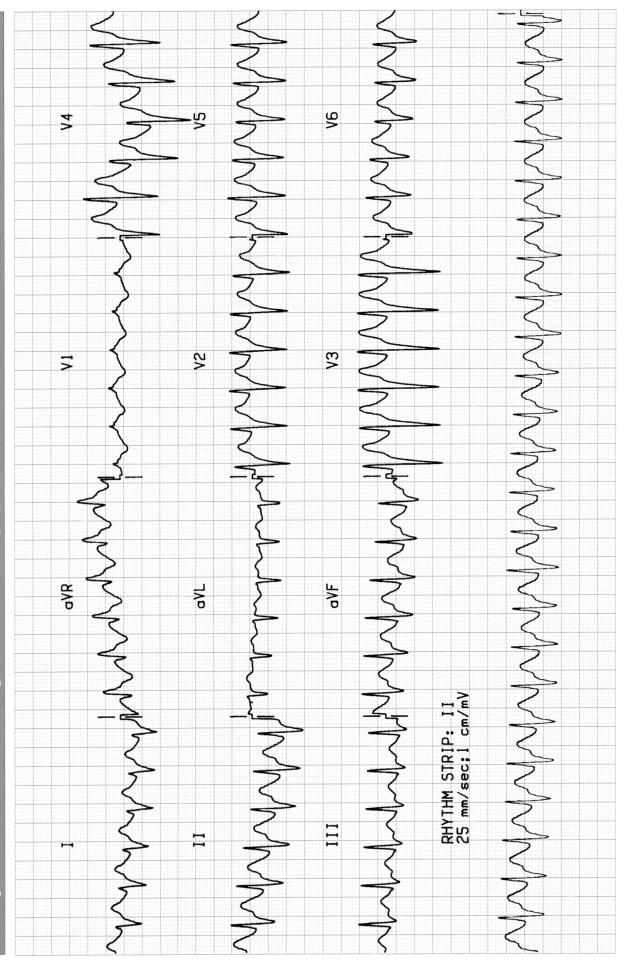

I

aVR

V1

V4

II

aVL

V2

V5

III

aVF

V3

V6

RHYTHM STRIP: II
25 mm/sec; 1 cm/mV

Tricyclic antidepressant overdose

- Sinus tachycardia.
- Long PR interval.
- Wide QRS.
- Long QT interval.
- A terminal 40 ms QRS axis of +120° to +270°.

FEATURES OF THIS ECG

- Indeterminate tachycardia, 145 b.p.m. (? sinus tachycardia, ? atrial flutter with 2:1 block)
- Features of tricyclic overdose (Fig. 74.1 and 74.2):
  - wide QRS (150 ms)
  - long corrected QT interval
  - Terminal 40 ms QRS axis deviation to the right suggested by an S in lead I and an R in lead aVR.

CLINICAL NOTE

This girl had taken 50 × 75 mg tablets of dothiepin.

A QRS duration of more than 100 ms is associated with an increased incidence of seizures and more than 160 ms with ventricular arrhythmias.[1] A terminal 40 ms QRS axis of 120–270°, in an overdose where the drug is not known, suggests tricyclic poisoning.[2]

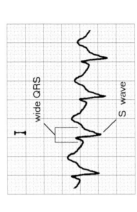

Fig. 74.1 Lead I.

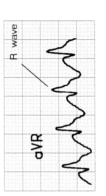

Fig. 74.2 Lead aVR.

Physical signs of tricyclic poisoning

- ↑ Dilated pupils
- ↑ Dry mouth
- ↑ Drowsiness
- ↑ Tachycardia
- ↑ Hypotension
- ↑ Urinary retention

[1] Boehnert M T, Lovejoy F H Jr 1985 Value of the QRS duration versus serum drug level in predicting seizures and ventricular arrhythmias after an acute overdose of tricyclic antidepressants. New England Journal of Medicine 313: 474–479
[2] Wolfe T R, Caravati E M, Rollins D E 1989 Terminal 40-ms frontal plane QRS axis as a marker for tricyclic antidepressant overdose. Annals of Emergency Medicine 18: 348–351

A 16-year-old boy with a history of 'faints'

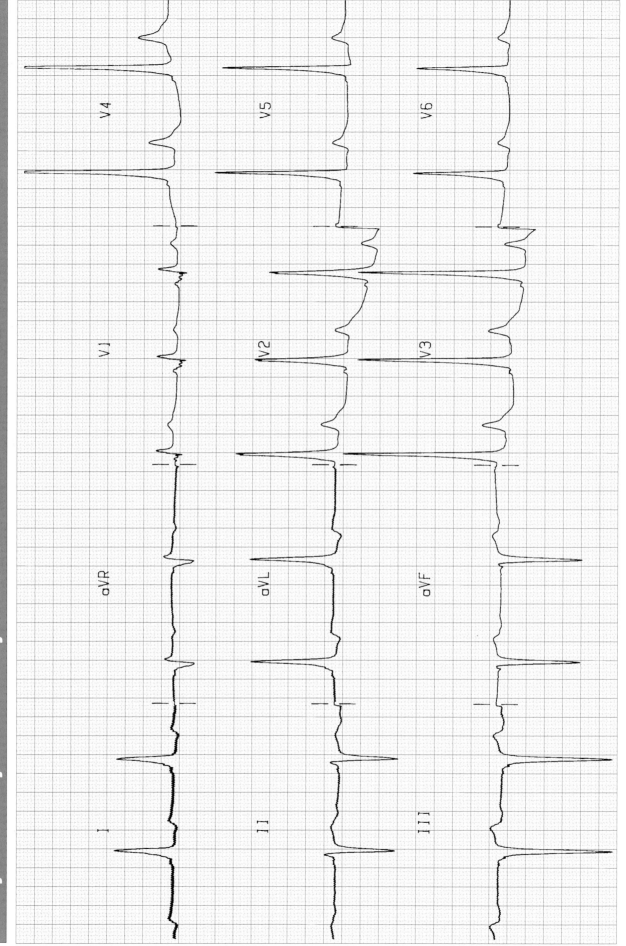

Wolf–Parkinson–White syndrome (1)

An accessory pathway (bundle of Kent) between the atria and ventricles may cause the following:

- short PR interval
- a delta wave of ventricular pre-excitation
- slightly widened QRS complex
- secondary ST and T wave changes
- a tendency to recurrent episodes of tachycardia.

CLINICAL NOTE

This is the recording of the same patient as on page 30 (WPW with AF).

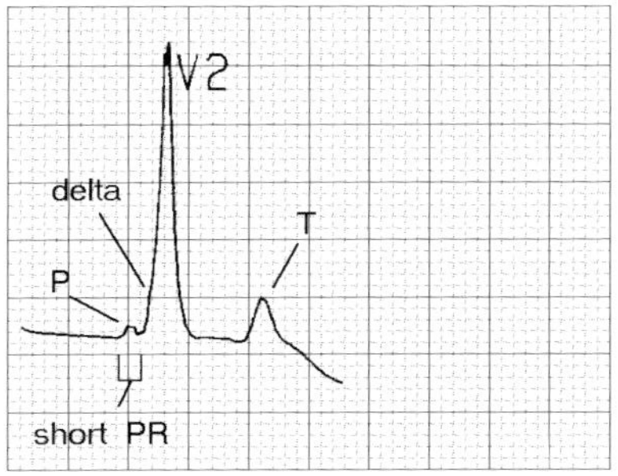

FEATURES OF THIS ECG

- Sinus rhythm, 60 b.p.m., left axis deviation –50°
- Features of Wolff–Parkinson–White syndrome (Fig. 75.1):
  - short PR interval
  - wide QRS
  - delta wave
- Secondary ST–T changes (Fig. 75.2)

The combination of left axis deviation and positive V1–3 suggests a left posteroseptal accessory pathway.

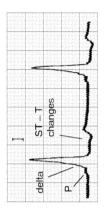

Fig. 75.1   Lead V2.

Fig. 75.2   Lead I.

WPW syndrome mimics other conditions

→ Right ventricular hypertrophy:
  - dominant R in lead V1
→ Myocardial infarction:
  - negative delta waves
  - ST–T changes
→ Bundle branch block:
  - delta wave appearing separate
→ Ventricular tachycardia:
  - antidromic AVRT

CASE 76

An 11-year-old boy with bouts of breathlessness

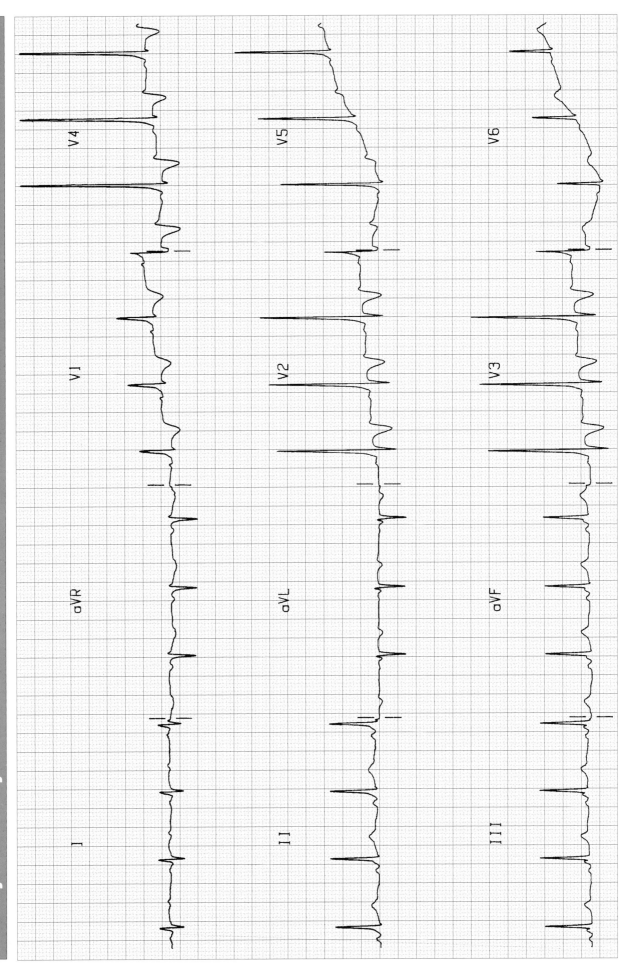

Wolff–Parkinson–White syndrome (2)

The commonest site for an accessory pathway is the left lateral region.

FEATURES OF THIS ECG

- Sinus rhythm, 84 b.p.m., vertical axis +90°
- Features of Wolff–Parkinson–White syndrome (Fig. 76.1):
  - short PR interval
  - wide QRS
  - delta wave
- Secondary ST–T changes (Fig. 76.2)

The combination of a rightward axis and positive V1–3 suggests a left lateral accessory pathway.

CLINICAL NOTE

This is the recording of the same patient as on page 26 (WPW orthodromic AV reciprocating tachycardia).

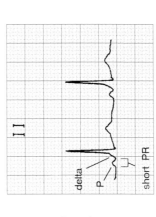

Fig. 76.1 Lead II.

Fig. 76.2 Lead V2.

Localising the accessory pathway

	V1	V2	QRS axis
Left posteroseptal (type A)	+ve	+ve	left
Right lateral (type B)	−ve	−ve	left
Left lateral (type C, commonest)	+ve	+ve	right
Right posteroseptal	−ve	+ve	left
Anteroseptal	−ve	−ve	normal

CASE 77

A routine preoperative recording

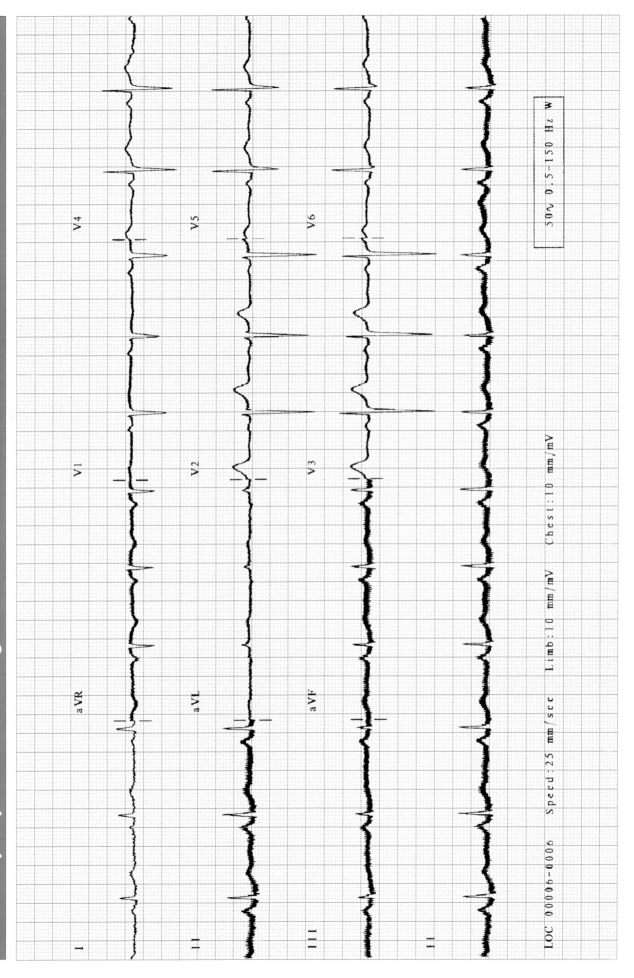

LOC 00006-0006   Speed:25 mm/sec   Limb:10 mm/mV   Chest:10 mm/mV

50~ 0.5-150 Hz W

Electrical interference

- A regular wave at 50–60 Hz superimposed on the recording.

FEATURES OF THIS ECG

- Sinus rhythm, 66 b.p.m., normal QRS axis
- Features of electrical interference (Fig. 77.1):
  – a regular wave thickening the baseline
- Otherwise normal recording

CLINICAL NOTE

Electrical interference is usually due to poor electrode contact, earthing problems or faulty equipment. It often distorts the finer detail of a recording.

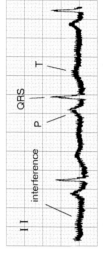

Fig. 77.1 Lead II.

CASE 78

A young man with non-specific chest pain

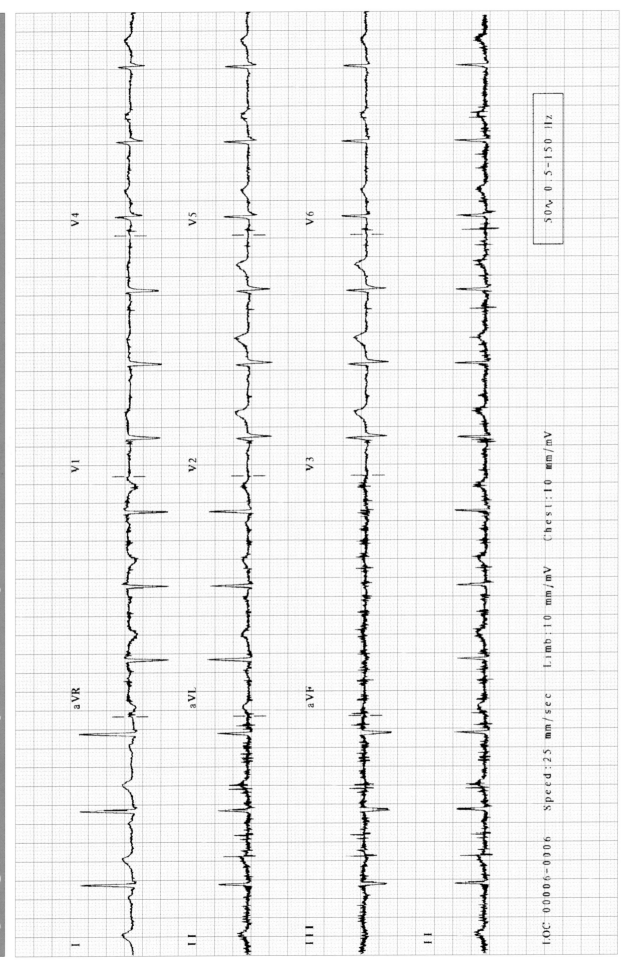

I

II

III

II

aVR

aVL

aVF

V1

V2

V3

V4

V5

V6

50~ 0.5-150 Hz

LOC: 00006-0006   Speed: 25 mm/sec   Limb: 10 mm/mV   Chest: 10 mm/mV

Skeletal muscle interference

- Irregular high frequency spikes of skeletal muscle contractions.

FEATURES OF THIS ECG

- Sinus rhythm, 72 b.p.m., normal QRS axis
- Features of skeletal muscle interference (Fig. 78.1):
  - high frequency spikes
- Otherwise normal recording

CLINICAL NOTE

Skeletal muscle interference is usually due to a nervous and tense patient. Ensure that the patient is calm with their head resting on a pillow and arms relaxed at each side. In a patient in pain or distress it is important to repeat the recording until the best possible trace is obtained.

Sometimes a regular skeletal muscle interference may be due to a tremor such as in Parkinson's disease.

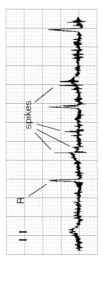

Fig. 78.1 Lead II.

CASE 79

A 50-year-old healthy man

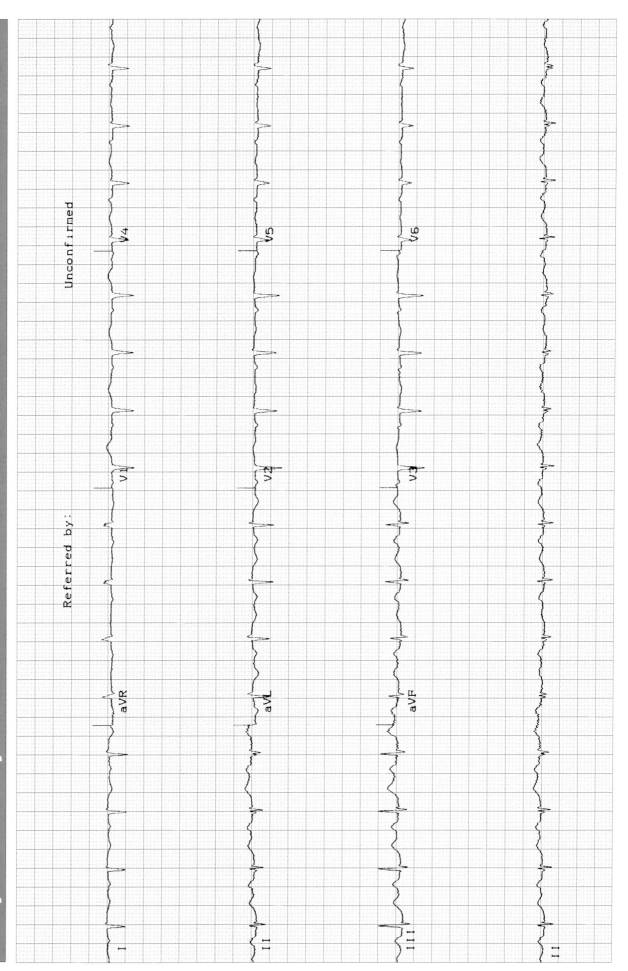

Unconfirmed

Referred by:

I
aVR
V1
V4

II
aVL
V2
V5

III
aVF
V3
V6

II

Dextrocardia

- Inverted P waves in lead I.
- Right axis deviation (usually).
- The QRS complexes get progressively smaller from V1 to V6.

FEATURES OF THIS ECG

- Sinus rhythm, 96 b.p.m., right axis deviation
- Features of dextrocardia:
  - inverted P wave in lead I (Fig. 79.1)
  - abnormal chest leads (Fig. 79.2):
    - (i) no R wave progression
    - (ii) QRS complexes becoming smaller from V1 to V6

CLINICAL NOTE

This man had dextrocardia and situs inversus.

To record a useful ECG in dextrocardia swap the left and right arm leads and place the chest leads in the same positions but swapped from left to right.

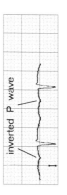

Fig. 79.1 Lead I.

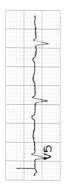

Fig. 79.2 Small R wave.

A 26-year-old medical student

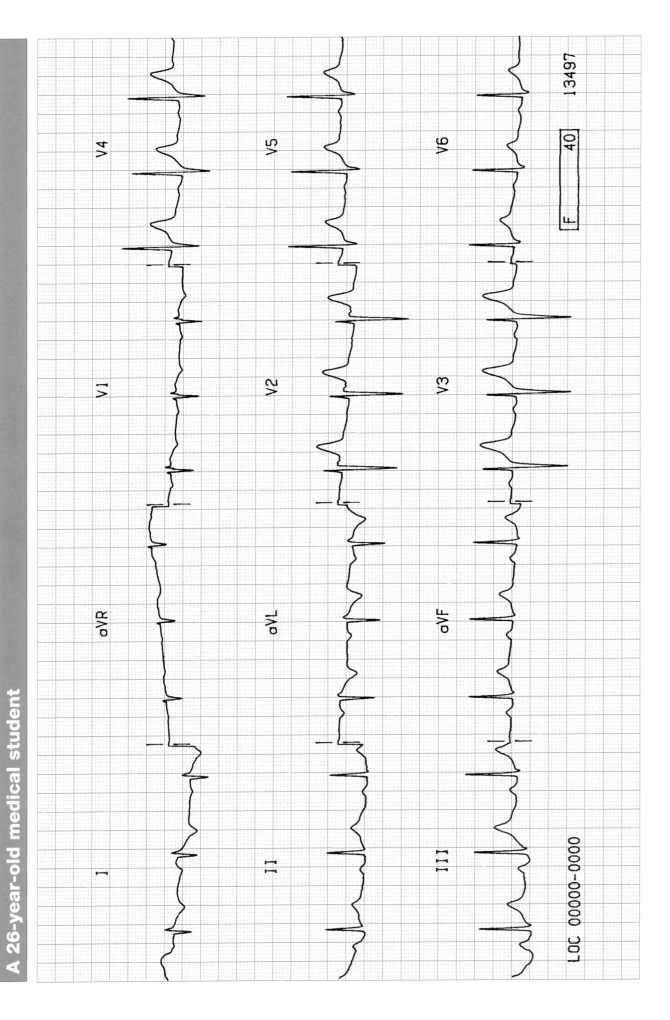

I

aVR

V1

V4

II

aVL

V2

V5

III

aVF

V3

V6

LOC 00000-0000

F 40

13497

'Technical' dextrocardia

- Inverted P waves in lead I.
- Right axis deviation (usually).
- Normal R wave progression in the chest leads.

'Technical' dextrocardia is produced by inadvertently swapping the leads for left and right arms. It is distinguished from true dextrocardia by the normal chest leads.

FEATURES OF THIS ECG

- Sinus rhythm, 72 b.p.m., right axis deviation
- Features suggesting 'technical' dextrocardia:
  - inverted P wave in lead I (Fig. 80.1)
  - right axis deviation (lead I negative)
  - normal appearance of the chest leads (Fig. 80.2)
- Incomplete right bundle branch block (Fig. 80.3):
  - rSr' pattern in lead V1
  - QRS duration less than 120 ms (three small squares)

CLINICAL NOTE

The effect of left–right arm lead reversal is a mirror image inversion of lead I, aVR swapped with aVL, lead II swapped with lead III and aVF unchanged.

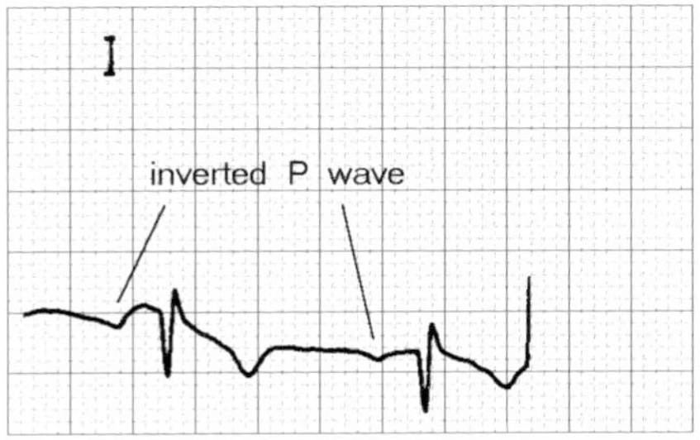

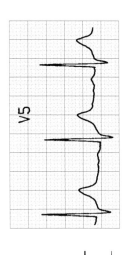

inverted P wave

I

Fig. 80.1 Lead I.

V5

Fig. 80.2 Normal R wave.

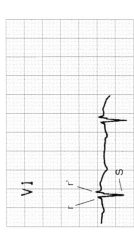

V1

r r'

s

Fig. 80.3 rSr' pattern.